An Atlas of

FETAL CENTRAL NERVOUS SYSTEM DISEASE

Diagnosis and Management

THE ENCYCLOPEDIA OF VISUAL MEDICINE SERIES

An Atlas of FETAL CENTRAL NERVOUS SYSTEM DISEASE

Diagnosis and Management

Ritsuko K. Pooh, MD, PhD

Department of Obstetrics and Maternal Fetal Medicine
National Kagawa Children's Hospital
Zentsuji, Kagawa, Japan

Kazuo Maeda, MD, PhD

Tottori University, Yonago and Seirei Hospitals
Hamamatsu, Shizuoka, Japan

KyongHon Pooh, MD

Department of Neurosurgery
National Kagawa Children's Hospital
Zentsuji, Kagawa, Japan

The Parthenon Publishing Group
International Publishers in Medicine, Science & Technology

A CRC PRESS COMPANY
BOCA RATON LONDON NEW YORK WASHINGTON, D.C.

Published in the USA by
The Parthenon Publishing Group
345 Park Avenue South, 10th Floor
New York
NY 10010
USA

Published in the UK and Europe by
The Parthenon Publishing Group
23–25 Blades Court
Deodar Road
London SW15 2NU
UK

Library of Congress Cataloging-in-Publication Data
Pooh, Ritsuko K.
An atlas of fetal central nervous system disease : diagnosis and management / Ritsuko K. Pooh, Kazuo Maeda, Kyong Hon Pooh.
p. ; cm. -- (The encyclopedia of visual medicine series)
Includes bibliographical references and index.
ISBN 1-84214-202-X (alk. paper)
1. Fetus--Diseases--Diagnosis--Atlases. 2. Central nervous system--Diseases--Diagnosis--Atlases. I. Maeda, Kazuo, 1925- II. Pooh, Kyong Hon. III. Title. IV. Series.
[DNLM: 1. Central Nervous System Diseases--diagnosis. 2. Fetal Diseases--diagnosis. WL 141 P821a 2003]
RG627.P66 2003
618.3'268--dc21 2003051291

British Library Cataloguing in Publication Data
Pooh, Ritsuko K.
An atlas of fetal central nervous system disease : diagnosis and management
1. Fetus - Diseases - Imaging. 2. Central nervous system - Diseases - Imaging
I. Title II. Maeda, Kazuo III. Pooh, KyongHon
618.3'268

ISBN 1-84214-202-X

First published in 2003

Composition by The Parthenon Publishing Group
Printed and bound by T. G. Hostench S.A., Spain

Contents

List of image contributors

Vincenzo D'Addario, MD, PhD
4th Unit Obstetrics and Gynecology
University Medical School
Bari, Italy

Shoichi Endo, MD, PhD
Department of Neurology
National Kagawa Children's Hospital
Kagawa, Japan

Kuniaki Fukuda, MD, PhD
Department of Neurology
National Kagawa Children's Hospital
Kagawa, Japan

Philippe Jeanty, MD, PhD
Women's Health Alliance
Department of Ultrasound
Nashville, USA

Ichiro Kawabata, MD, PhD
Department of Obstetrics and Gynecology
Gifu University School of Medicine
Gifu, Japan

Yoshimasa Kinoshita, MD
Department of Neurosurgery
Munakata Suikokai General Hospital
Fukuoka, Japan

Gustavo Malinger, MD
Prenatal Diagnosis Unit
Department of Obstetrics and Gynecology
Edith Wolfson Medical Center
Holon, Israel

Koreaki Mori, MD, PhD
Kochi Medical School
Kochi, Japan

Takeshi Murakoshi, MD, PhD
Department of Obstetrics and Gynecology
Seirei Hamamatsu General Hospital
Shizuoka, Japan

Yoshinobu Nakagawa, MD, PhD
Department of Neurosurgery
National Kagawa Children's Hospital
Kagawa, Japan

Kouhei Shiota, MD, PhD
Department of Anatomy and Developmental Biology
Kyoto University Faculty of Medicine
Kyoto, Japan

Mitsuyo Tanemura, MD, PhD
Department of Obstetrics and Gynecology
Nagoya City University
Nagoya, Japan

Masaji Utsu, MD, PhD
Department of Obstetrics and Gynecology
Seirei Mikatahara General Hospital
Shizuoka, Japan

Hidetsuna Utsunomiya, MD, PhD
Department of Radiology
Fukuoka University
Fukuoka, Japan

Renato Ximenes, MD
Centrus – Ultrasound and Fetal Medicine
Campinas, Brazil

Nobuhiro Yamamoto, MD
Department of Obstetrics and Gynecology
Fujinomiya Municipal Hospital
Shizuoka, Japan

Preface

The central nervous system (CNS) is the most attractive and important organ. During fetal life, the brain and spinal cord are rapidly formed from their premature appearance into a mature systematic organ. Various phenotypes of CNS abnormalities, including congenital anomalies and brain injuries *in utero,* arise as a result of insults which can occur in the early, middle or late stages of pregnancy. Advanced neuroimaging technology such as transvaginal sonography, three-dimensional ultrasound and magnetic resonance imaging have revealed these various CNS abnormalities and have provided a natural history *in vivo* of the abnormalities, opening up a new era in prenatal diagnosis and management. This Atlas has been written for easy understanding of advanced neuroimaging technologies, accurate CNS diagnosis *in utero*, and obstetric and postnatal neurosurgical management of fetal CNS diseases.

Ritsuko Kimata Pooh

Acknowledgements

We would like to express our great appreciation to GE Medical Systems (Milwaukee, USA) and Kretztechnik (Zipf, Austria) for their technical support of three- and four-dimensional ultrasound technology, and clinical collaborative cooperation. We also thank Mr Yoshihiko Nagao for his skillful work in magnetic resonance imaging, and all image contributors for their very sophisticated and comprehensive images and schemas. Lastly, we greatly appreciate the fetuses who have taught and shown us the truth *in utero*.

1

Background and role of fetal central nervous system: diagnosis and management

R.K. Pooh

BACKGROUND OF FETAL CENTRAL NERVOUS SYSTEM ASSESSMENT

In utero neuroimaging of anomalies

Recent advances in prenatal imaging technologies, such as transvaginal ultrasound, three-dimensional ultrasound and magnetic resonance imaging (MRI), have been remarkable and have contributed to the prenatal evaluation of fetal abnormalities *in utero*. Owing to these technologies, fetal malformations have been reliably diagnosed with increasing accuracy and at an earlier gestation. As for the fetal central nervous system (CNS) assessment, a new field of 'neurosonography'[1] has been established. Many congenital CNS anomalies, which were disclosed in late pregnancy or after birth, have been demonstrated recently by use of high-frequency transvaginal sonography before viability. More advances in technological development will clarify unknown neuropathological facts during the fetal period.

Neonatal encephalopathy

In terms of encephalopathy or cerebral palsy, 'timing of the brain insult, antepartum, intrapartum or postpartum' is one of the serious controversial issues including medico–socio–legal–ethical problems. Although brain insults may relate to antepartum events in a substantial number of term infants with hypoxic–ischemic encephalopathy, the timing of the insult cannot always be clarified. It is a hard task to give antepartum evidence of brain injury predictive of cerebral palsy. Fetal heart rate monitoring cannot reveal the presence of encephalopathy, and neuroimaging by ultrasound and MRI is the most reliable modality for disclosure of silent encephalopathy. Many cases of cerebral palsy with acquired brain insults, especially in term infants with reactive fetal heart rate tracing and good Apgar scores at delivery, are not suspected of having encephalopathy and are often overlooked for months or years. Recent imaging technology has demonstrated cases with brain insult *in utero*.

Difficulties of fetal CNS assessment

Diagnostics of the fetal CNS is one of the most difficult fields in perinatology. There are several reasons why the prenatal CNS evaluation is difficult:

(1) Lack of essential knowledge of CNS anatomy and pathology (see Chapter 2);

(2) Rapid changes of normal CNS development during pregnancy (see Chapter 2);

(3) Inexperience of CNS neuroimaging techniques (see Chapter 3).

When beginners start prenatal CNS imaging, these three points may be the most frequent reasons for difficulties in prenatal assessment. However, after overcoming those problems, there still exist difficulties in assessment of fetal CNS diseases:

(1) Difficulty in prediction of neurological prognosis;

(2) Existence of a gray zone between normality and abnormality.

It is extremely hard to make a neurological prognosis by abnormal morphology. Figure 1.1 shows the comparison before and after treatment in cases with hydrocephalus or porencephaly. The prognosis is good in both cases despite abnormal morphology

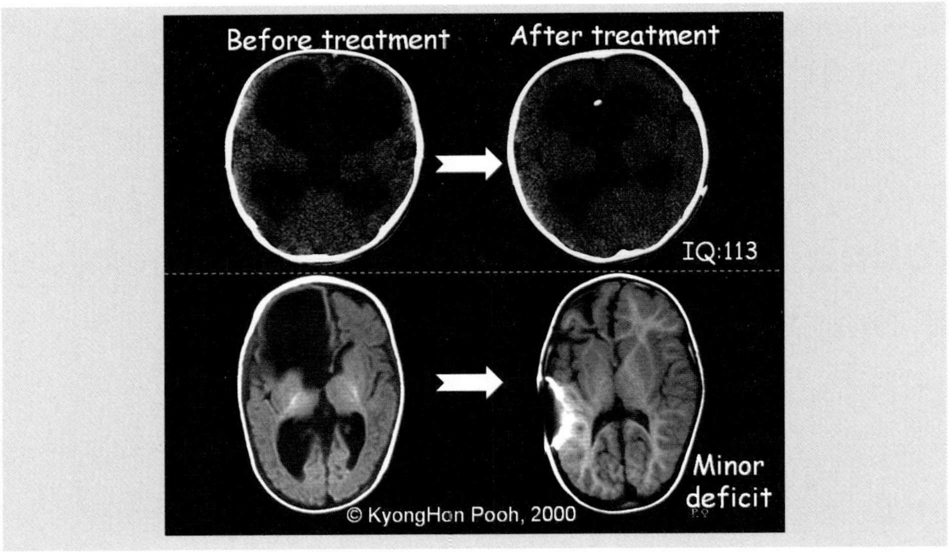

Figure 1.1 Abnormal morphology and neurological prognosis. Upper, a case of hydrocephalus. After treatment by a shunt operation, ventriculomegaly still exists. However, this infant has developed normally with an IQ of 113. Lower, a case of progressive ventriculomegaly with a porencephalic cyst. After treatment, ventriculomegaly and porencephaly resolved but the brain morphology is not complete. This case has had an almost normal postoperative course with very subtle motor disturbance. The morphology does not always correspond to the neurological prognosis

even after treatment. Morphology does not always correspond to the neurological prognosis. One more cause which makes prenatal evaluation difficult is the existence of a gray zone between normality and abnormality.

ROLE OF FETAL CENTRAL NERVOUS SYSTEM DIAGNOSIS

The initial purpose of prenatal neuroimaging is to confirm normal CNS development with advancing gestation. Second, the role of neuroimaging is to detect abnormalities with accuracy and objectivity for proper perinatal management and care. Once abnormal findings of the fetal brain and/or spine are suspected, counselling the parents should be carried out prudently. Ambiguous or uncertain diagnoses make parents overanxious and may lead them to an overhasty decision since the 'CNS' may preside over important parts of fetal life and may also influence the lives of the rest of the family. In particular, a fetal CNS diagnosis before viability should be performed precisely and prudently. The more accurate and objective the diagnosis, the better the parents understand and carefully consider the facts presented to them about their unborn fetus. Drotar and colleagues[2] analyzed interviews with parents of neonates with congenital malformations disclosed at birth, and proposed five stages of parental reactions:

- Shock
- Denial
- Sadness and anger
- Adaptation
- Reorganization

We interviewed mothers of neonates with congenital malformations diagnosed *in utero* who were repeatedly well-informed during pregnancy, and analyzed maternal psychological changes. When fetal anomalies were disclosed, denial, sadness, guilt and anxiety arose in the mothers' minds. By the time of delivery, however, most of the mothers accepted the fact of having congenitally malformed babies (Figure 1.2). Moreover, when the mothers first faced their newborn babies, most of them were relieved and decided to cherish their babies (Figure 1.3). These mothers had already reached Drotar's last stage of 'reorganization' at birth. Thus, prenatal diagnosis and subsequent serial counselling during pregnancy play an important role in leading parents with unborn malformed babies to the stages of adaptation and reorganization.

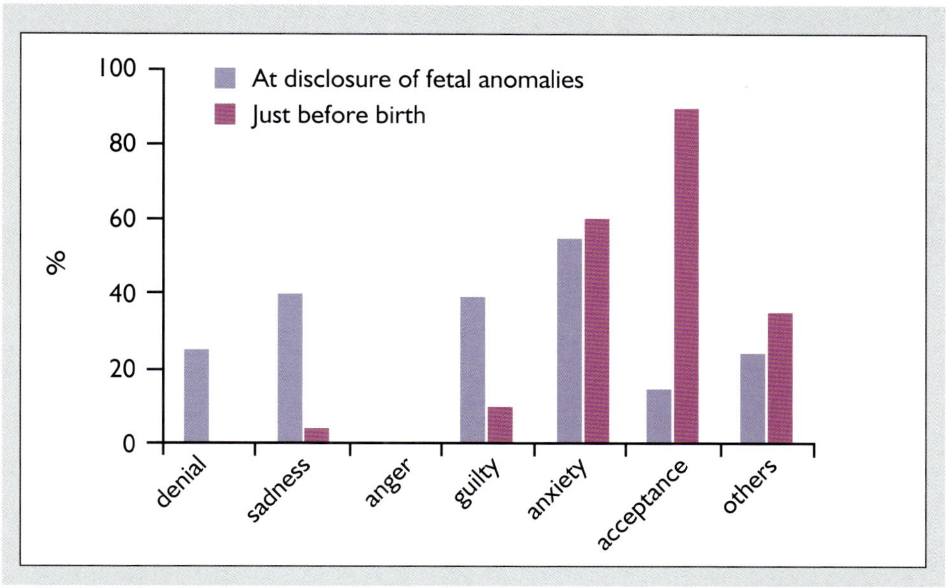

Figure 1.2 Comparison of the mental state in mothers who have fetal congenital malformations disclosed *in utero* between the time of disclosure of fetal anomalies and just before birth

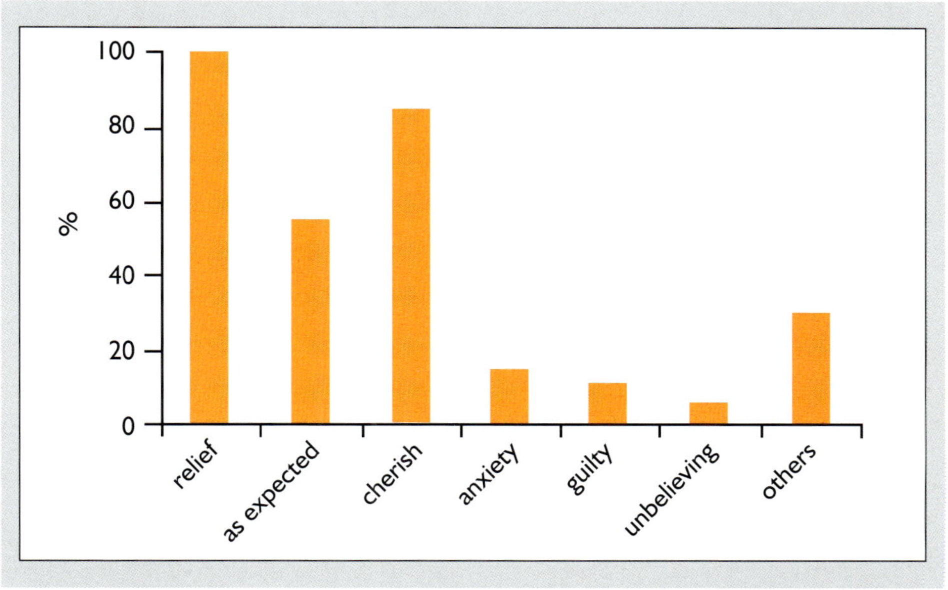

Figure 1.3 Mental state just after delivery in mothers who have fetal congenital malformations disclosed *in utero*

REFERENCES

1. Timor-Tritsch IE, Monteagudo A. Transvaginal fetal neurosonography: standardization of the planes and sections by anatomic landmarks. *Ultrasound Obstet Gynecol* 1996;8:42–7

2. Drotar D, Baskiewicz A, Irvin N, *et al*. The adaptation of parents to the birth of an infant with a congenital malformation: a hypothetical model. *Pediatrics* 1975;56:710–17

2

Central nervous system development and anatomy

R.K. Pooh

CENTRAL NERVOUS SYSTEM DEVELOPMENT

The brain is a three-dimensional structure and should be studied in the three orthogonal views of sagittal, coronal and axial section (Figure 2.1). During the fetal period, the embryonal premature CNS structure develops into the mature structure (Figures 2.2–2.9). Within this rapid change of development, various developmental disorders and/or insults result in various phenotypes of fetal CNS abnormalities. For understanding fetal CNS diseases, basic knowledge of the development of the nervous system is essential. The developmental stages and their major disorders (see Chapter 6) are described in Table 2.1.

BASIC KNOWLEDGE OF BRAIN ANATOMY FOR NEUROIMAGING

It may be believed by many that the anatomy of the brain must be complicated and therefore there must be a large number of terms to remember. In this Chapter, essential anatomical structures have been selected for neuroimaging and the comprehension of fetal CNS diseases. Figures 2.10 and 2.11 show the sagittal and anterior coronal sections of the brain. For understanding hydrocephalus, ventriculomegaly and/or other intracranial lesions, the ventricular system (Figure 2.12) and cerebral spinal fluid (CSF) circulation (Figure 2.13) should be understood.

Table 2.1 Developmental stages and major disorders

Developmental stage	*Disorders*
Primary neurulation (3–4 weeks' gestation)	spina bifida aperta, cranium bifidum
Caudal neural tube formation (secondary neurulation, from 4 weeks' gestation)	occult dysraphic states
Prosencephalic development (2–3 months' gestation)	holoprosencephaly, agenesis of the corpus callosum, agenesis of the septum pellucidum, septo-optic dysplasia
Neuronal proliferation (3–4 months' gestation)	micrencephaly, macrencephaly
Neuronal migration (3–5 months' gestation)	schizencephaly, lissencephaly, pachygyria, polymicrogyria
Organization (5 months' gestation to years postnatal)	idiopathic mental retardation
Myelination (birth to years postnatal)	cerebral white matter hypoplasia

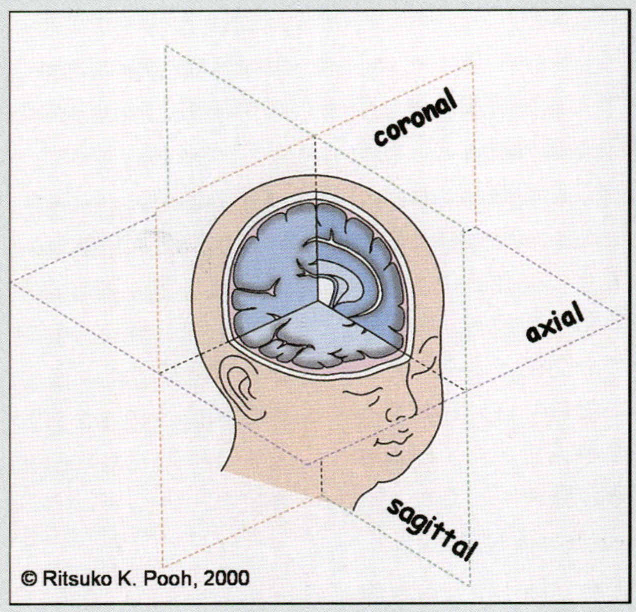

Figure 2.1 Basic three orthogonal sections of the brain. For easy understanding of brain anatomy and neuroimaging, these three sections are fundamental

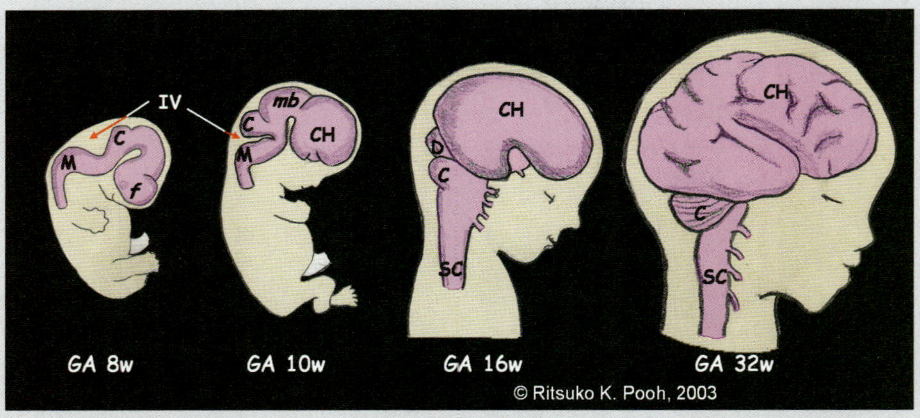

Figure 2.2 Developing brain and spinal cord during pregnancy. The fetal central nervous system changes in size and appearance from an early premature structure into a late mature structure with gyral formation. CH, cerebral hemisphere; C, cerebellum; D, diencephalon; M, medulla; SC, spinal cord; f, forebrain; mb, midbrain; IV, fourth ventricle; GA, gestational age

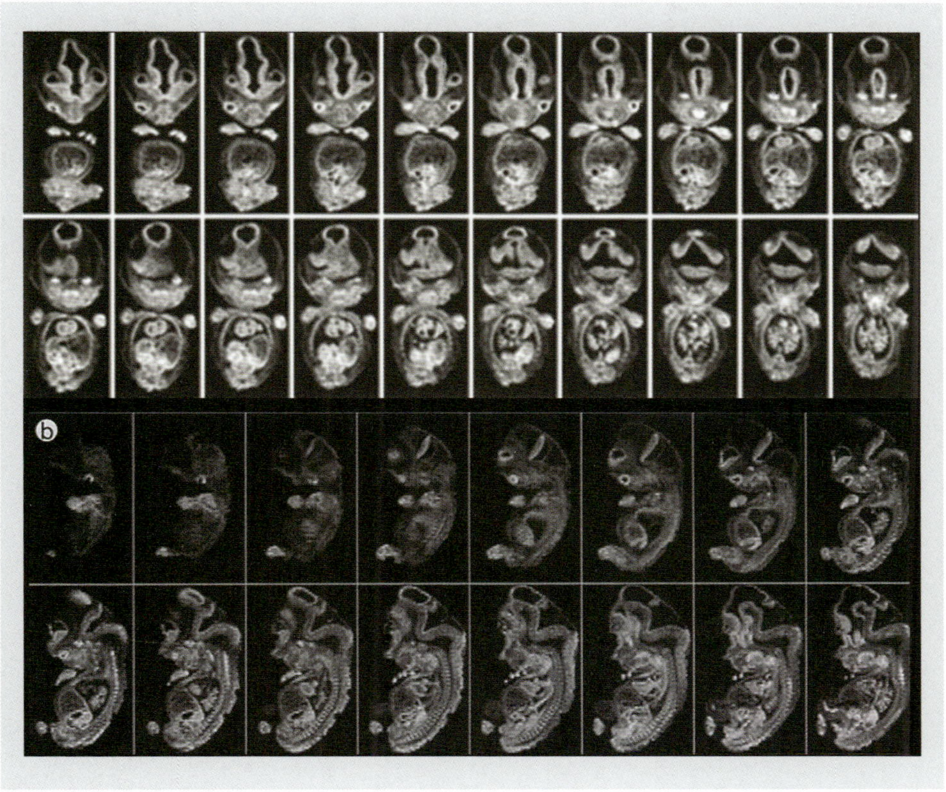

Figure 2.3 Serial magnetic resonance images (MRI) of early fetus (7 weeks of gestation). Upper, serial coronal MRI of the fetus at 7 weeks' gestational age. Lower, serial sagittal MRI of the fetus at 7 weeks' gestational age. Germinal matrix cannot be detected. Image contributed by Dr Kinoshita, from *AJNR* 2001;22:382 and *Clinical Imagiology* 2001;17:1392, with permission

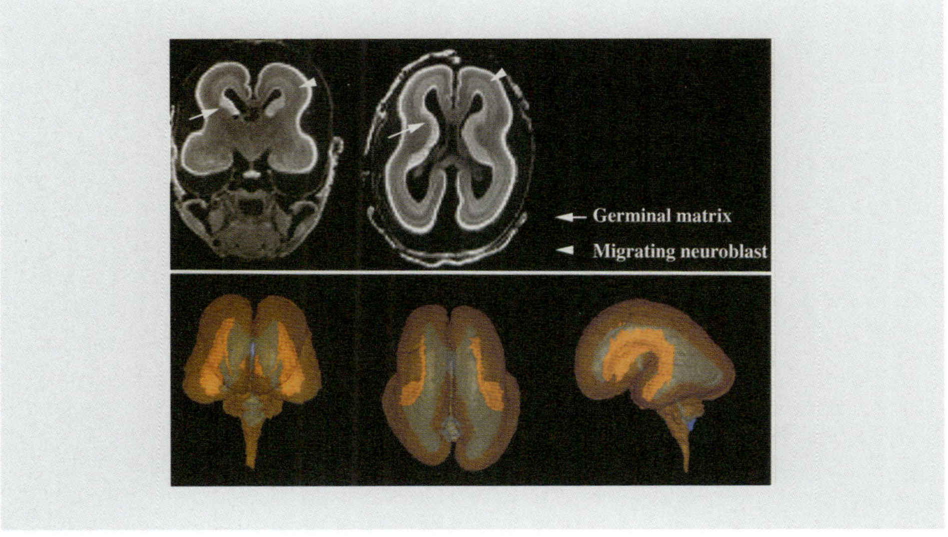

Figure 2.4 Magnetic resonance sectional images and magnetic resonance surface-rendering images of a stillborn infant at 21 weeks of gestation. Note the germinal matrix (arrow) and migrating neuroblast (arrowhead). In the lower figures, the ventricular system is demonstrated in blue and the germinal matrix in orange. Image courtesy of Dr Kinoshita, from *Jap J Clin Radiol* 1999;44:1235, with permission

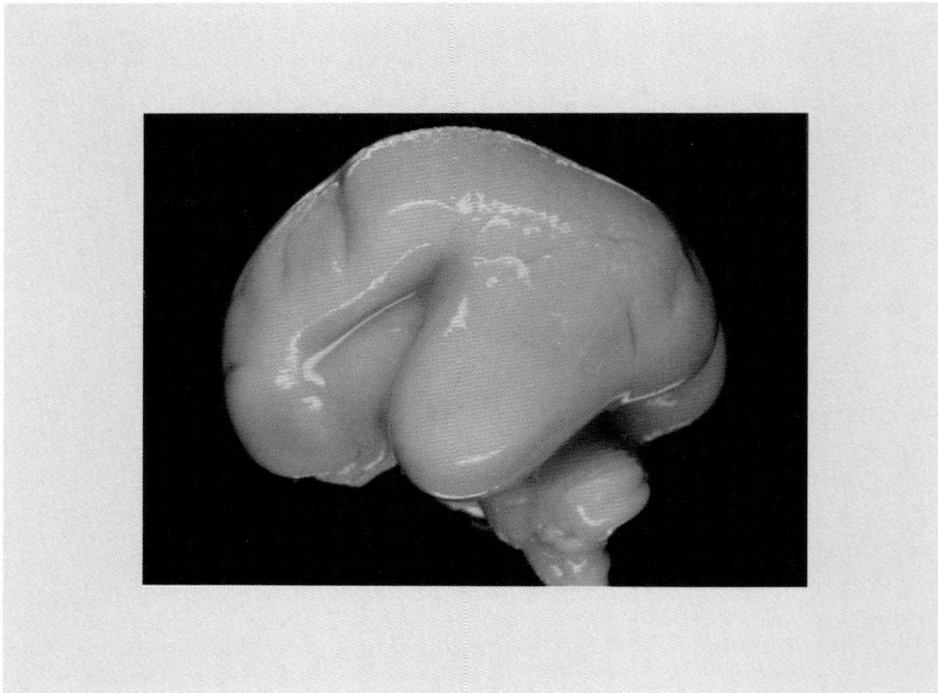

Figure 2.5 Photomicrograph of a lateral view of the brain of a stillborn fetus (20 weeks, crown–rump length 170 mm). From Moore KL, Persaud TVN and Shiota K. *Color Atlas of Clinical Embryology*. 2nd edn, Philadelphia: W.B. Saunders, 2000, with permission. Specimen was from Congenital Anomaly Research Center, Kyoto University Graduate School of Medicine

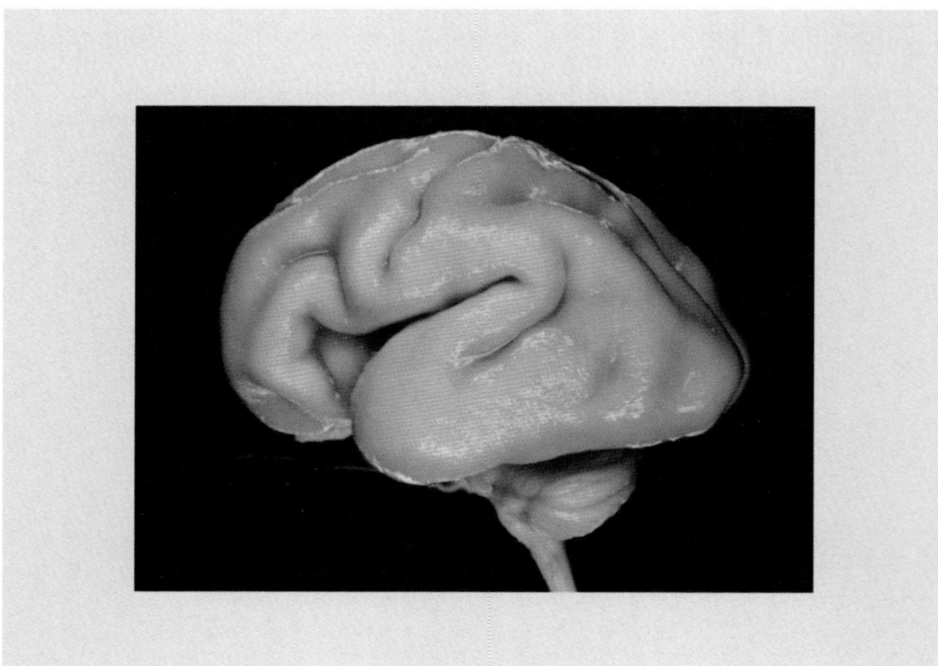

Figure 2.6 Photomicrograph of a lateral view of the brain of a stillborn fetus (25 weeks). From Moore KL, Persaud TVN, Shiota K. *Color Atlas of Clinical Embryology*. 2nd edn. Philadelphia: W.B. Saunders, 2000, with permission. Specimen was from the Congenital Anomaly Research Center, Kyoto University Graduate School of Medicine

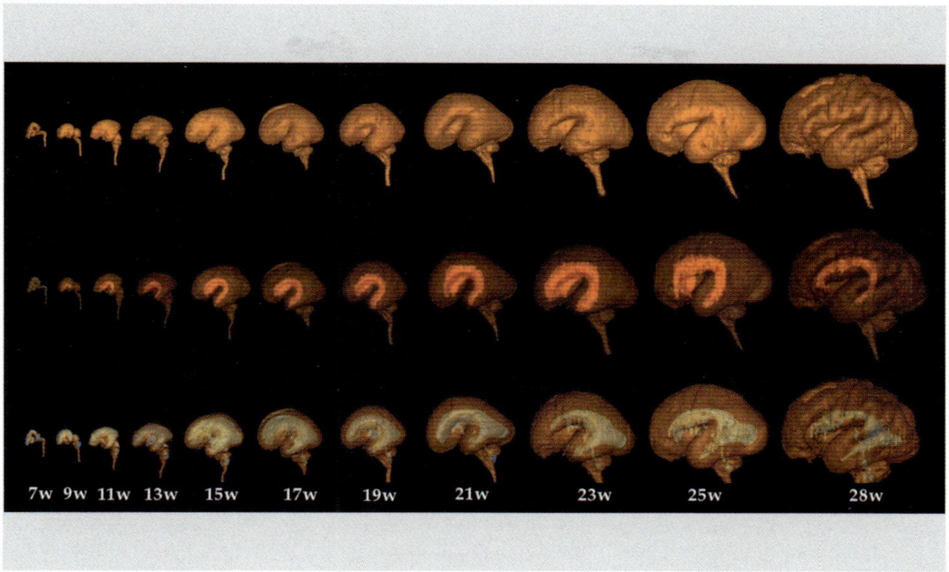

Figure 2.7 Three-dimensional reconstruction magnetic resonance images (MRI) of the brain surface, germinal matrix and ventricular system. Successive MRIs of stillborn fetuses show developmental changes in the lateral configuration of the brain, germinal matrix and ventricular system. The brain surfaces (upper row), germinal matrix (middle row, orange) and ventricular system (lower row, blue) of human fetal brain were reconstructed by surface rendering. The volume of the germinal matrix increased until 23 weeks' gestational age and decreased rapidly at 28 weeks' gestational age. Note how the lateral ventricles change from fetal type, with vesicular aspect and bicornuate shape, to adult type with increasing gestational age. Image courtesy of Dr Kinoshita, from *AJNR* 2001;22:382, with permission

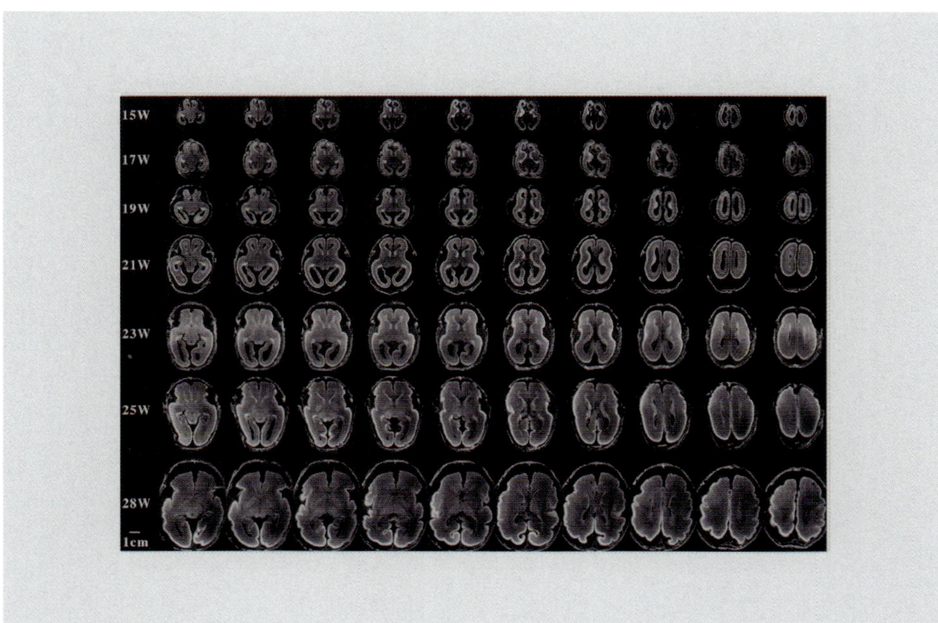

Figure 2.8 Serial axial magnetic resonance images (MRI) of postmortem stillborn fetuses between 15 and 28 weeks of gestation. Note the lateral ventricular change from fetal type, with vesicular aspect and bicornuate shape, to adult type. Image courtesy of Dr Kinoshita, from *Clinical Imagiology* 2001;17:1392, with permission

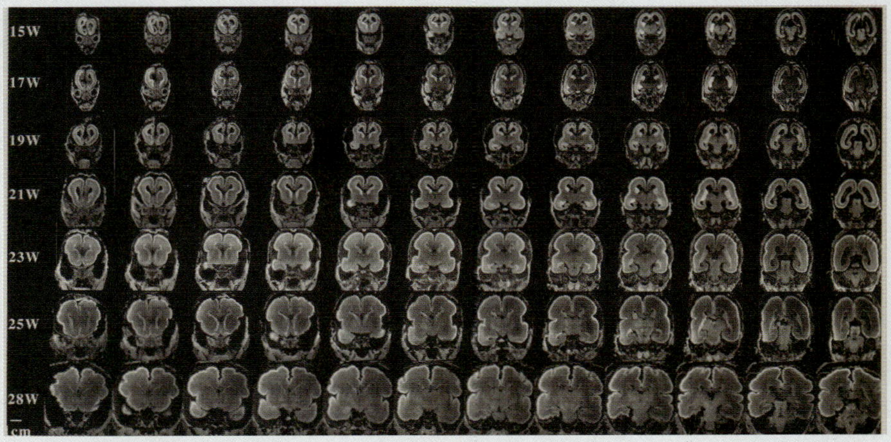

Figure 2.9 Serial coronal magnetic resonance images of stillborn fetuses between 15 and 28 weeks of gestation. Note the lateral ventricular change from fetal type, with vesicular aspect and bicornuate shape, to adult type. Image courtesy of Dr Kinoshita, from *Clinical Imagiology* 2001;17:1392, with permission

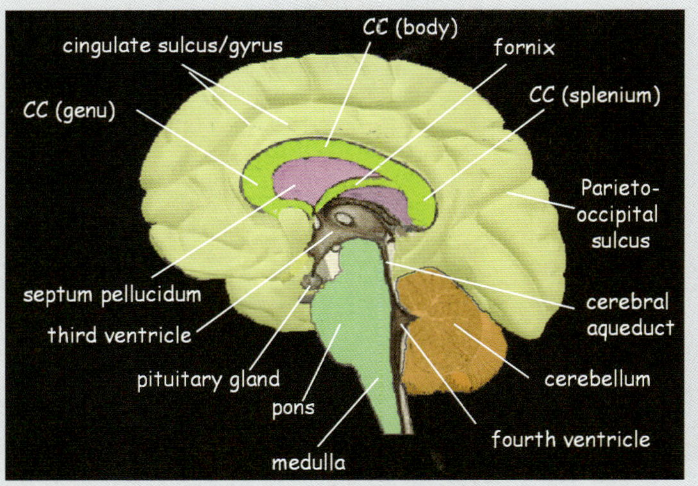

Figure 2.10 Basic anatomical structure of sagittal cutting section of the brain. CC, corpus callosum

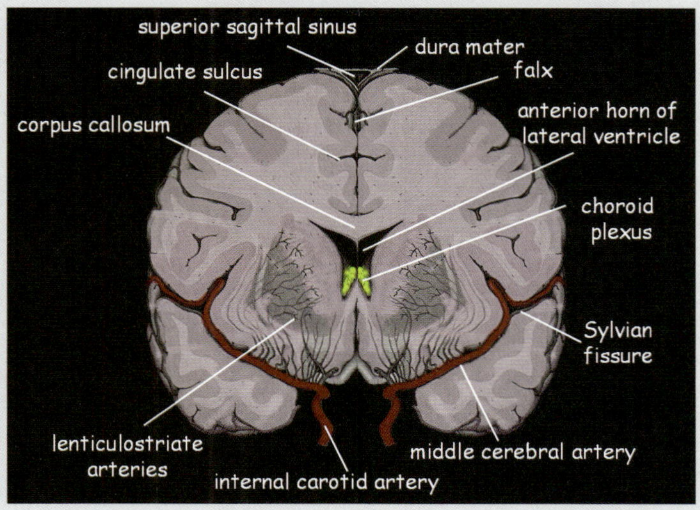

Figure 2.11 Basic anatomical structure of coronal cutting section of the brain

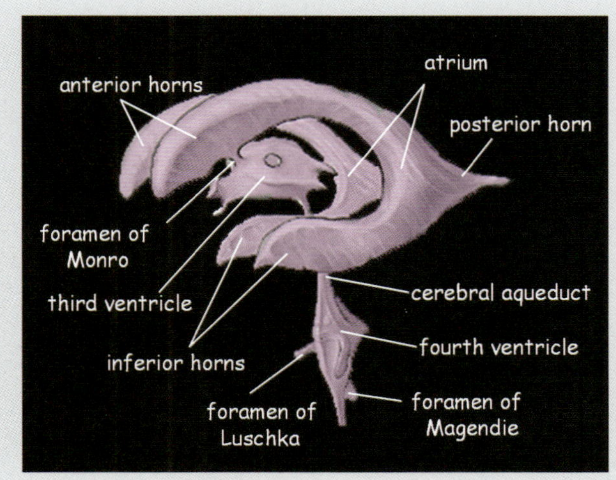

Figure 2.12 Basic anatomical structure of the ventricular system of the brain. Cerebrospinal fluid (CSF), produced from the choroid plexus of the ventricles, runs from the lateral ventricles, through the third ventricle, aqueduct, fourth ventricle and goes to the surface of the brain and spinal cord

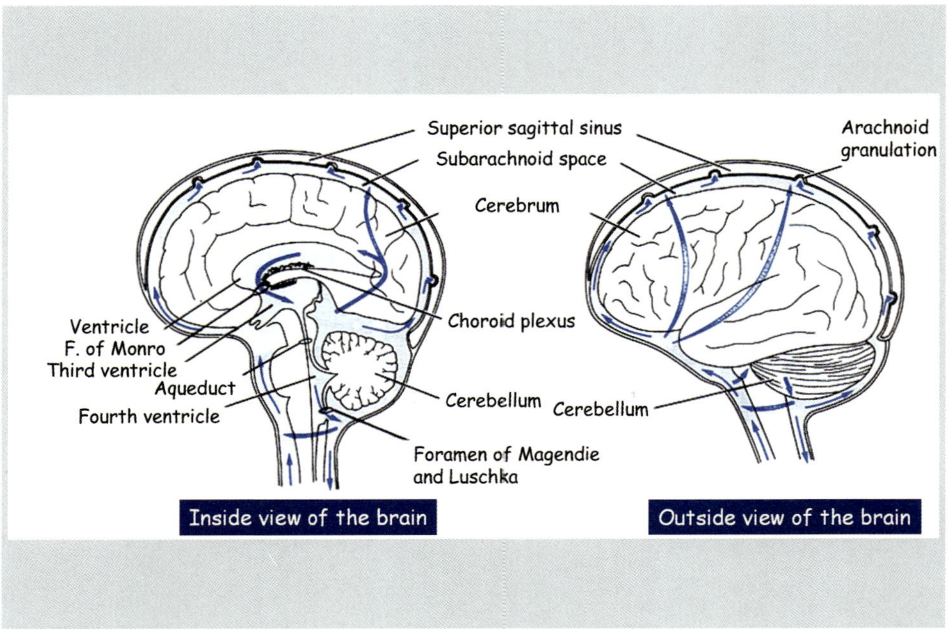

Figure 2.13 Cerebrospinal fluid (CSF) circulation. Inside and outside views of the brain. CSF is produced from the choroid plexus of the ventricles. CSF runs through the third ventricle, aqueduct and fourth ventricle, to the surface of the brain and spinal cord, and is then absorbed by arachnoid granulation. From *Handbook on Hydrocephalus for Patients*, Research Committee of 'Intractable Hydrocephalus', Japanese Ministry of Health and Welfare, ©1993, with permission. Schema courtesy of Chairman of the Committee, Professor K. Mori

3

Technologies and techniques of fetal neuroimaging diagnosis

R.K. Pooh and K. Maeda

TRANSABDOMINAL SONOGRAPHY

The transabdominal sonographic technique (Figure 3.1), by which it is possible to observe the fetal internal organs through the maternal abdominal wall and uterine wall, has been the most widely used for fetal imaging diagnosis. By using the transabdominal approach, the fetal brain structure, mainly in the axial section, and fetal back structure including the vertebrae and spinal cord in the sagittal section, can be well demonstrated. However, when using the transabdominal approach to the fetal central nervous system, there are several obstacles, such as the maternal abdominal wall, the placenta and the fetal cranial bones.

TRANSVAGINAL SONOGRAPHY

The introduction of the high-frequency transvaginal transducer has contributed to establishing 'sonoembryology'[1] and the recent general use of

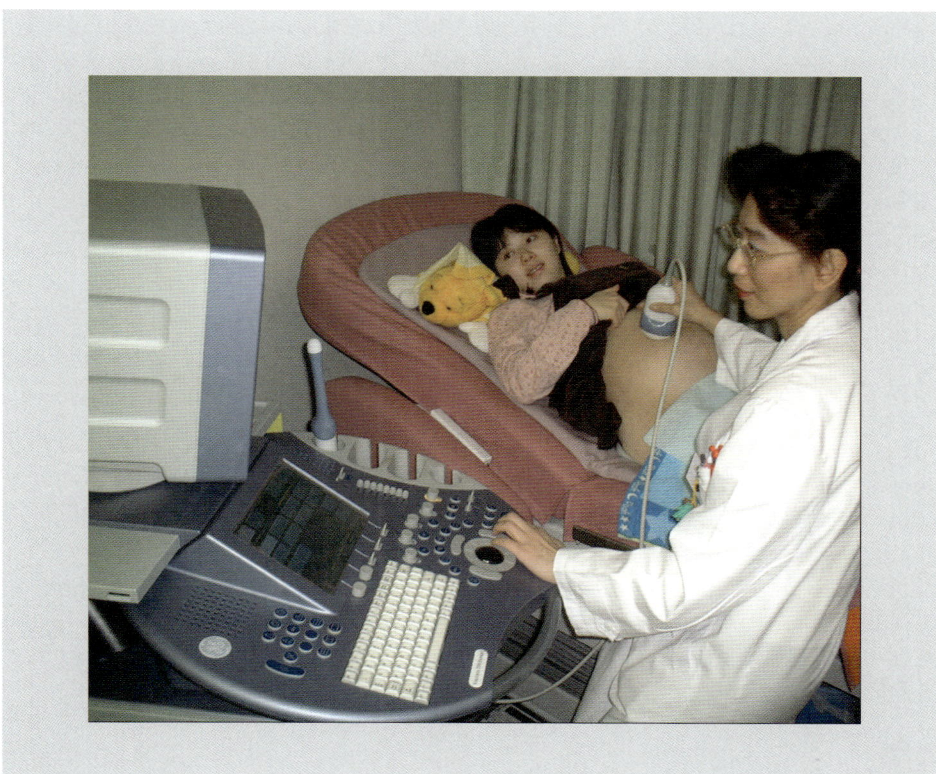

Figure 3.1 Transabdominal sonography for fetal central nervous system imaging

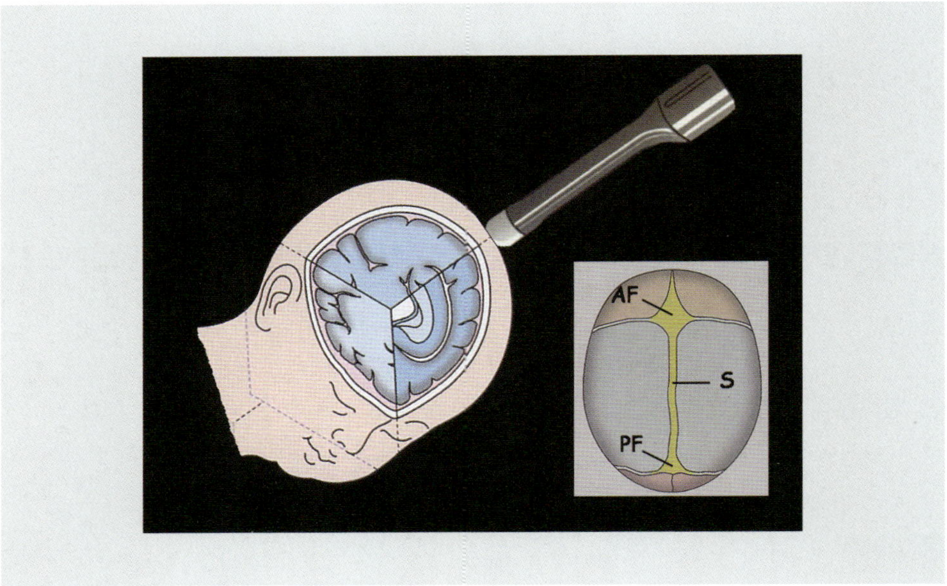

Figure 3.2 Transvaginal approach to the fetal brain and the ultrasound windows. Transvaginal sonography enables demonstration of the sagittal and coronal planes of the brain. The anterior fontanelle (AF), sagittal suture (S) and posterior fontanelle (PF) are ultrasound windows for approaching the brain

transvaginal sonography in early pregnancy has enabled the early diagnosis of major fetal anomalies[2]. In middle and late pregnancy, the fetal CNS is generally evaluated through the maternal abdominal wall. By using transabdominal sonography, the fetal brain is mainly demonstrated in transcranial axial sections. The brain, however, is a three-dimensional structure, and should be assessed in the basic three planes, sagittal, coronal and axial sections (Figure 2.1). Sonographic assessment of the fetal brain in the sagittal and coronal sections, requires an approach from the fetal parietal direction (Figure 3.2). Transvaginal sonography of the fetal brain (Figures 3.3 and 3.4) opened up a new field in medicine, 'neurosonography'[3]. The transvaginal approach to the normal fetal brain during the second and third trimester was introduced at the beginning of the 1990s. It was the first practical application of three-dimensional central nervous system assessment by two-dimensional ultrasound[4]. Transvaginal observation of the fetal brain offers sagittal and coronal views of the brain from the fetal parietal direction[5–8] through the fontanelles and/or the sagittal suture as ultrasound windows. Serial oblique sections[3] via the same ultrasound window reveal the intracranial morphology in detail. This method has contributed to the prenatal assessment of congenital CNS anomalies and acquired brain damage *in utero*.

THREE-DIMENSIONAL ULTRASOUND

Three-dimensional ultrasound is one of the most attractive modalities in the field of fetal ultrasound imaging. There are two scanning methods – the free-hand scan and the automatic scan. The automatic scan by dedicated three-dimensional transducer produces motor-driven automatic sweeping and is called a fan scan (Figure 3.5). With this method, a shift and/or angle change of the transducer is not required during scanning and scan duration is only a few seconds. After acquisition of the target organ, multiplanar imaging analysis is possible. The combination of both transvaginal sonography and three-dimensional ultrasound[9–12] may be a great diagnostic tool for evaluation of the three-dimensional structure of the fetal CNS. There are several useful functions in three-dimensional ultrasound as shown below:

(1) Surface imaging of the fetal head;
(2) Bony structural imaging of the calvaria and vertebrae;
(3) Multiplanar imaging of the intracranial structure;
(4) Three-dimensional sonoangiography of the brain circulation;

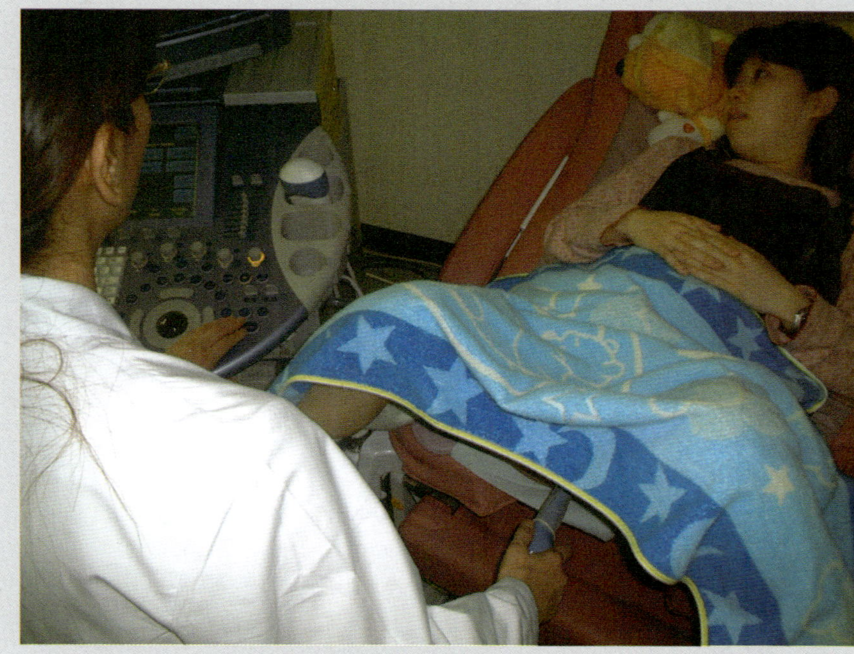

Figure 3.3 Transvaginal sonography for fetal central nervous system imaging

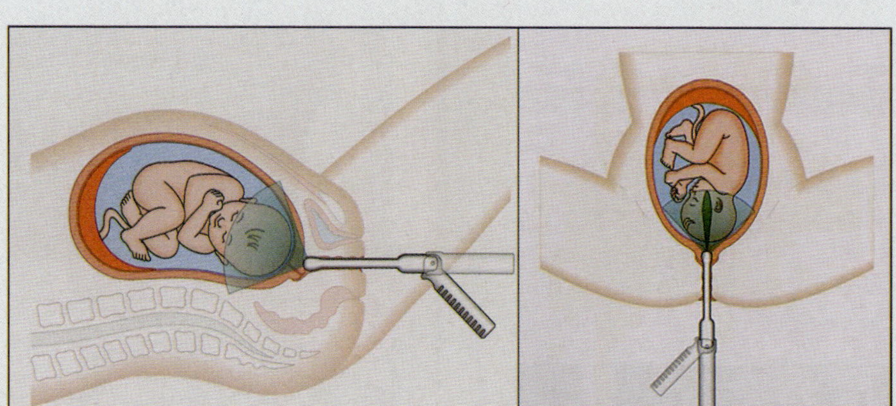

Figure 3.4 Schema of transvaginal sonography. Left, lateral view of vertex-presenting fetus and transvaginal transducer. Right, frontal view. Clear imaging is possible by rotating and angle changing of the transducer

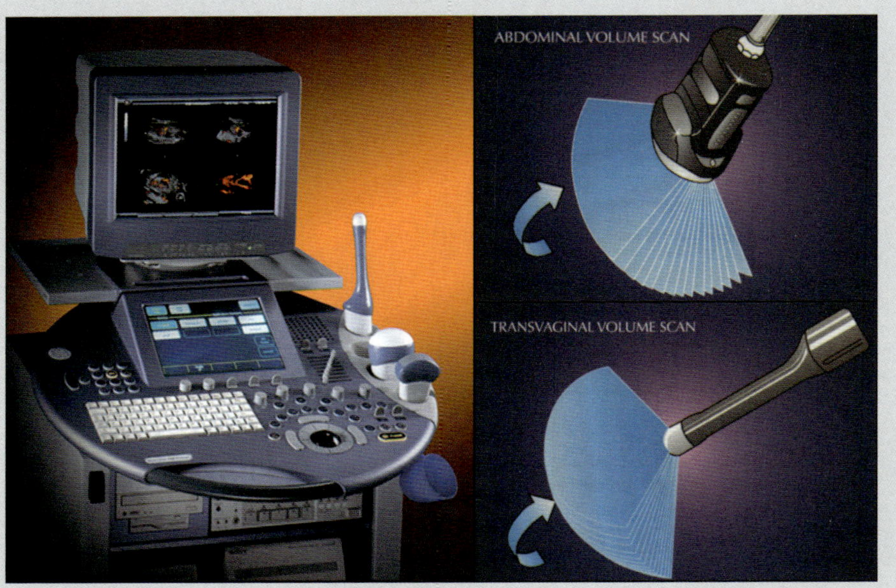

Figure 3.5 Device and transducers for three-dimensional and four-dimensional ultrasound. Three-dimensional ultrasound provides not only surface imaging but also multiplanar inner structural analysis, vascular analysis and volumetric analysis. A recent advance in three-dimensional ultrasound has introduced four-dimensional ultrasound with volume contrast imaging. Picture and schemas courtesy of GE Medical Systems and Kretztechnik

(5) Volume calculation of target organs such as the intracranial cavity, ventricle, choroid plexus and intracranial lesions;

(6) Simultaneous volume contrast imaging by four-dimensional ultrasound.

In multiplanar imaging of the brain structure, it is possible to demonstrate not only the sagittal and coronal sections but also the axial section of the brain (Figure 3.6), which cannot be demonstrated from the parietal direction by conventional two-dimensional transvaginal sonography. Parallel slicing provides tomographic visualization of internal morphology similar to MRI. Volume-extracted images and volume calculation of the fetal brain in early pregnancy were reported in the 1990s[13,14]. We used transvaginal three-dimensional ultrasound and the 3D View version 3.2 software (Kretztechnik AG, Zipf, Austria) for volume extraction and volume estimation of the brain structure (Figure 3.7). Furthermore, with the application of four-dimensional ultrasound, real-time images with increased contrast resolution can be obtained not only in the same plane as the two-dimensional cutting section but also in a vertical plane to the two-dimensional image[15].

Fetal neuroimaging with advanced three- and four-dimensional technology is an easy, non-invasive and reproducible method. It produces not only comprehensible images but also objective imaging data which can be graphed in volume calculation. Easy storage/extraction of a raw volume dataset enables off-line analysis and consultation with neurologists and neurosurgeons[16,17].

ULTRASONIC TISSUE CHARACTERIZATION BY GRAY-LEVEL HISTOGRAM WIDTH

Ultrasonic B-mode usually diagnoses the morphology of the tissue, organ or mass, while for some diagnostic purposes, echogenicity plays an important role. For example, periventricular echodensity (PVE), which is discussed later in this atlas, is defined by its higher echogenicity than that of the choroid plexus. The diagnosis is usually made by visual observation of the ultrasound image, but it is a

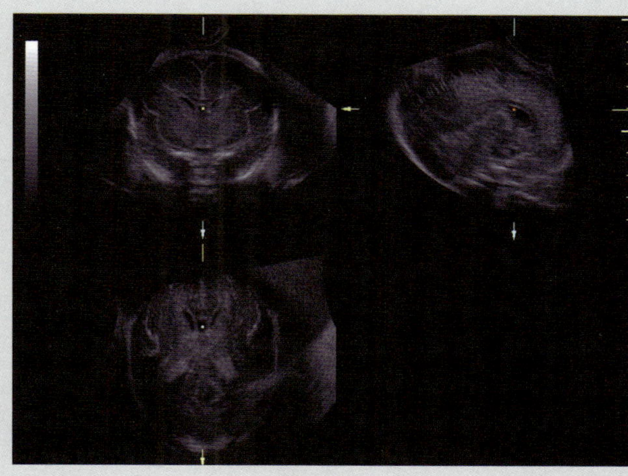

Figure 3.6 Three-dimensional multiplanar image analysis. Three orthogonal views are useful to obtain orientation of the brain structure. The raw three dimensional volume dataset can be saved quickly. Saved data can be reviewed on the ultrasound device, and extracted on CD-R(W) or MO disks and sent for consultation. Off-line image analysis can be carried out easily and repeatedly

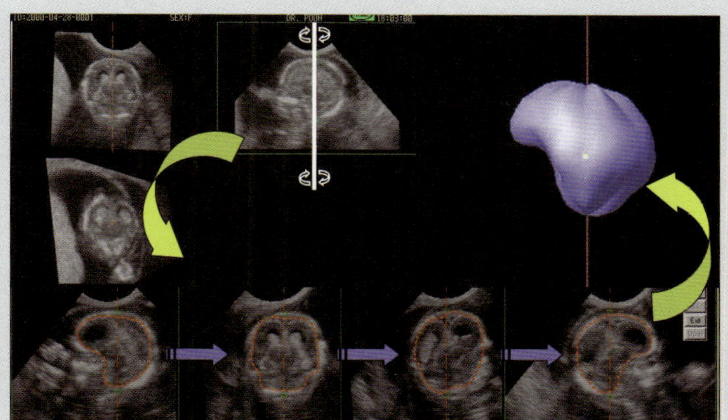

Figure 3.7 Three-dimensional volume extraction and volumetric analysis. On three orthogonal sections, the target organ can be traced automatically or manually by rotation of the volume imaging data. After tracing, a volume extraction image (upper right) can be demonstrated and volume calculation data are shown. Three-dimensional volumetry adds objective graphed imaging data

subjective decision. A more objective method is required for scientific analysis. Many tissue characterization techniques have been reported for this purpose, but most of them need particular algorithms, special software, and often sophisticated computers, which are difficult to supply in many general hospitals. The gray-level histogram width (GLHW; Figure 3.8) for clinical tissue characterization, is based on the measurement of the width of the gray-level histogram. This can be is displayed on

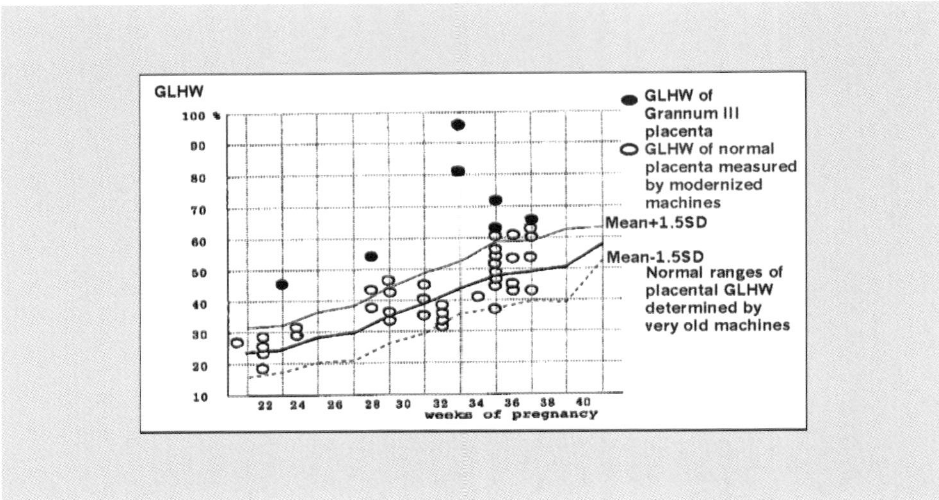

Figure 3.8 Examples of gray-level histogram width (GLHW). GLHW in a normal placenta every 2 weeks during pregnancy and a large GLHW in a Grannum III placenta[18]. There is no influence of the device and image depth on the GLHW in studies on ultrasound phantoms. Only its increase is calibrated in high image contrast[1]. The GLHW is high in a Grannum III placenta[18], in fetal periventricular echodensity[21], in meconium-stained fluid, in ovarian malignancy and endometrial cancer, while it is low in the immature fetal lung[19,20]

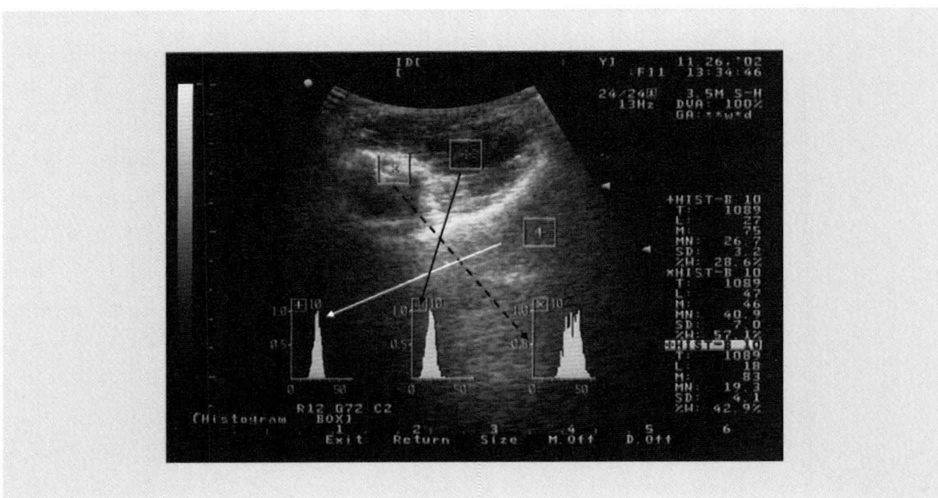

Figure 3.9 Procedures for the detection of an ultrasound histogram using a common imaging device. 1. Usual scan using a common commercial machine, or with a two-dimensional histogram from a Kretz three-dimensional machine. 2. Freeze the display of the subject image on the screen, press 'USER', select a region of interest (ROI) on the panel, and place it at the tissue image. Select 'HISTO' shape and size from the menu, if necessary. 3. Pixel gray levels in the ROI are processed for the histogram and data analysis. These are displayed on the screen as shown in the Figure

the image of a common commercial ultrasound imaging device (Figure 3.9) and, also, on the screen of a three-dimensional machine and, in addition, it needs no particular computer or software for its measurement. The GLHW is not influenced by the device gain or by the image depth, and needs only easy calibration when the image contrast is high. The manual technique is usual, while automated

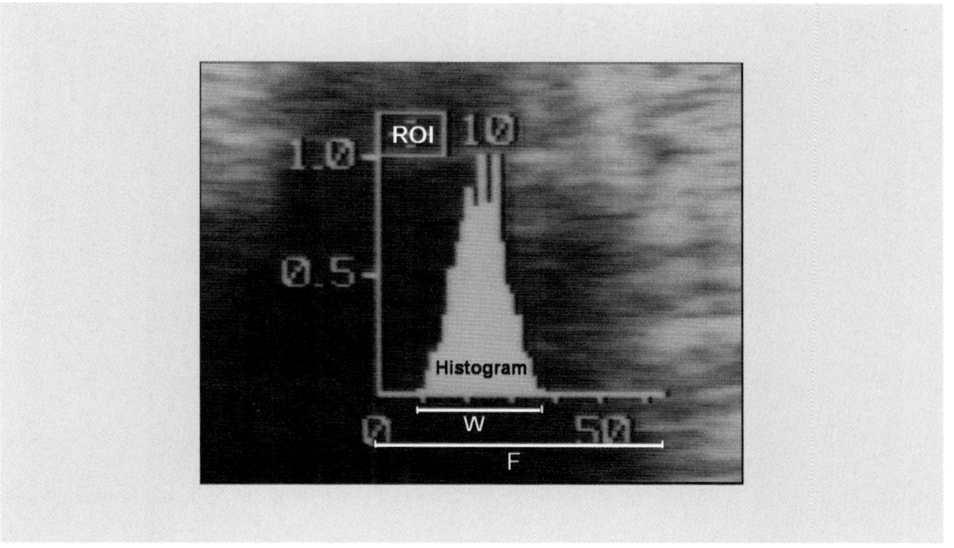

Figure 3.10 Determination of gray-level histogram width (GLHW) on the ultrasonic image. GLHW = (W/F) x 100 (%). ROI, region of interest; histogram, frequency histogram of pixel gray levels in the ROI; W, base width of the histogram; F, full gray-scale length. The automated GLHW provided by Aloka (Tokyo, Japan) was identical to the manual determination

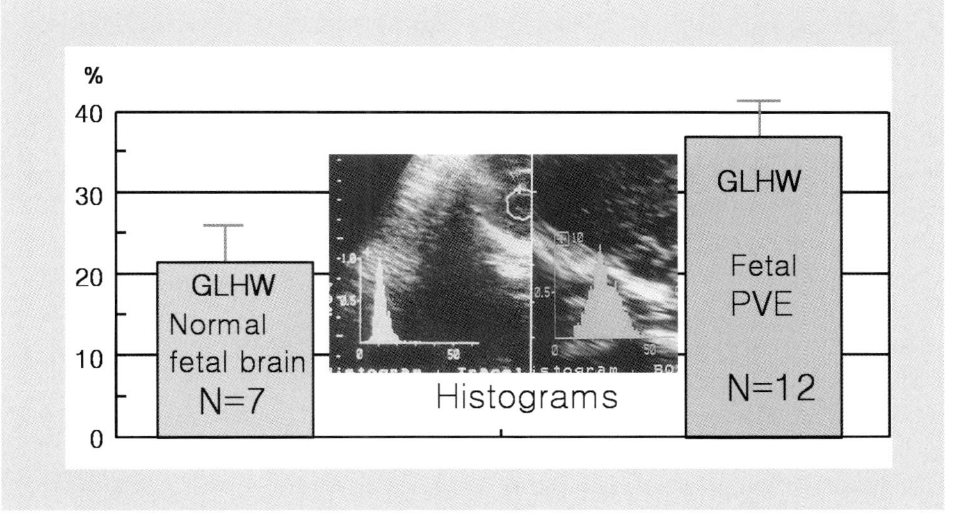

Figure 3.11 An example of the gray-level histogram width (GLHW) application in the fetal central nervous system: objective detection of fetal periventricular echodensity (PVE). The histogram is wider and the GLHW is larger in a fetal PVE image than in that of a normal fetal brain. Twin peaks appear in some PVE histograms. Image courtesy of Dr N. Yamamoto

measurement is also provided as an option[18,19] (Figure 3.10). High Grannum-grade placenta, immature fetal lung, meconium-stained amniotic fluid, ovarian masses, endometial cancer and other conditions have been diagnosed by GLHW, in addition to fetal cerebral PVE[20,21] (Figure 3.11).

MAGNETIC RESONANCE IMAGING

Recently, MRI has frequently been used in the obstetric field for maternal and fetal imaging diagnosis. In particular, fast MRI is being used increasingly as a correlative imaging modality because it uses no

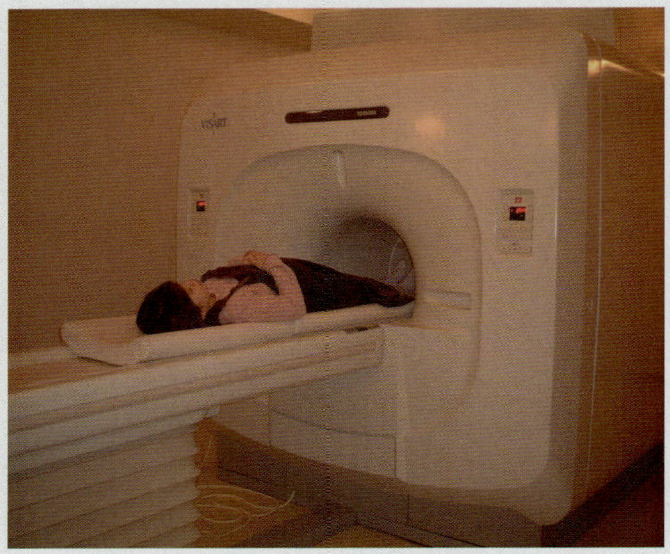

Figure 3.12 Magnetic resonance imaging of the fetus

ionizing radiation, provides excellent soft tissue contrast, has multiple planes for reconstruction, and a large field of view[22]. Recent advances in fast MRI technology, such as half-Fourier and the 0.5-signal-acquired single-shot fast spin-echo (SE), half-Fourier rapid acquisition with relaxation enhancement (RARE) sequences, has remarkably improved the T2-weighted image resolution despite a short acquisition time, and has minimized fetal and/or maternal respiratory motion artifacts without need of fetal sedation[23]. MRI has great potential especially for the evaluation of CNS and several reports have been published on normal and abnormal CNS anatomy by using fast MRI techniques[24–28]. In this atlas, we have used a 1.5 T MR unit with two-dimensional half-Fourier fast SE sequence (Figure 3.12) for assessment of fetal CNS abnormalities. Before MRI, sonographic localization of the organ of interest is performed. The most suitable coil is selected and set according to the maternal position and location of the target organ. MRI demonstrates the brain structure in detail, including the brainstem which cannot be clearly depicted even by transvaginal sonography. In cases with CNS abnormalities, which should be operated on immediately after birth, detailed prenatal information is quite helpful and does not require postnatal neuroimaging before an initial treatment.

REFERENCES

1. Timor-Tritsch IE, Peisner DB, Raju S. Sonoembryology: an organ-oriented approach using a high-frequency vaginal probe. *J Clin Ultrasound* 1990;18:286–98

2. Pooh RK. B-mode and Doppler studies of the abnormal fetus in the first trimester. In Chervenak FA, Kurjak A, eds. *Fetal Medicine*. Carnforth, UK: Parthenon Publishing, 1999:46–51

3. Timor-Tritsch IE, Monteagudo A. Transvaginal fetal neurosonography: standardization of the planes and sections by anatomic landmarks. *Ultrasound Obstet Gynecol* 1996;8:42–7

4. Monteagudo A, Reuss ML, Timor-Tritsch IE. Imaging the fetal brain in the second and third trimesters using transvaginal sonography. *Obstet Gynecol* 1991;77:27–32

5. Monteagudo A, Timor-Tritsch IE, Moomjy M. *In utero* detection of ventriculomegaly during the second and third trimesters by transvaginal sonography. *Ultrasound Obstet Gynecol* 1994;4:193–8

6. Monteagudo A, Timor-Tritsch IE. Development of fetal gyri, sulci and fissures: a transvaginal sonographic study. *Ultrasound Obstet Gynecol* 1997;9:222–8

7. Pooh RK, Nakagawa Y, Nagamachi N, *et al.* Transvaginal sonography of the fetal brain: detection of abnormal morphology and circulation. *Croat Med J* 1998;39:147–57

8. Pooh RK, Maeda K, Pooh KH, *et al.* Sonographic assessment of the fetal brain morphology. *Prenat Neonat Med* 1999;4:18–38

9. Pooh RK. Three-dimensional ultrasound of the fetal brain. In Kurjak A, ed. *Clinical Application of 3D Ultrasonography.* Carnforth, UK: Parthenon Publishing, 2000:176–80

10. Pooh RK, Pooh KH, Nakagawa Y, *et al.* Clinical application of three-dimensional ultrasound in fetal brain assessment. *Croat Med J* 2000;41:245–51

11. Timor-Tritsch IE, Monteagudo A, Mayberry P. Three-dimensional ultrasound evaluation of the fetal brain: the three horn view. *Ultrasound Obstet Gynecol* 2000;16:302–6

12. Monteagudo A, Timor-Tritsch IE, Mayberry P. Three-dimensional transvaginal neurosonography of the fetal brain: 'navigating' in the volume scan. *Ultrasound Obstet Gynecol* 2000;16:307–13

13. Blaas HG, Eik-Nes SH, Kiserud T, *et al.* Three-dimensional imaging of the brain cavities in human embryos. *Ultrasound Obstet Gynecol* 1995;5:228–32

14. Blaas HG, Eik-Nes SH, Berg S, *et al. In-vivo* three-dimensional ultrasound reconstructions of embryos and early fetuses. *Lancet* 1998;352:1182–6

15. Pooh RK, Pooh KH. Fetal neuroimaging with new technology. *Ultrasound Rev Obstet Gynecol* 2002;2:178–81

16. Pooh RK, Pooh KH. Transvaginal 3D and Doppler ultrasonography of the fetal brain. *Semin Perinatol* 2001;25:38–43

17. Pooh RK, Pooh KH. The assessment of fetal brain morphology and circulation by transvaginal 3D sonography and power Doppler. *J Perinat Med* 2002;30:48–56

18. Maeda K, Utsu M, Kihaile PE. Quantification of sonographic echogenicity with gray level histogram width: a clinical tissue characterization. *Ultrasound Med Biol* 1998;24:225–34

19. Maeda K, Utsu M, Yamamoto N, *et al.* Echogenicity of fetal lung and liver quantified by the gray-level histogram width. *Ultrasound Med Biol* 1999;25:201–8

20. Maeda K, Utsu M, Yamamoto N, *et al.* Clinical tissue characterization with gray level histogram width in obstetrics and gynecology. *Ultrasound Rev Obstet Gynecol* 2002;2:124–8

21. Yamamoto N, Utsu M, Maeda K, *et al.* Neonatal periventricular leukomalacia preceded by fetal periventricular echodensity. *Fetal Diag Ther* 2000;15:198–208

22. Levine D. Magnetic resonance imaging in prenatal diagnosis. *Curr Opin Pediatr* 2001;13:572–8

23. Huisman TA, Wisser J, Martin E, *et al.* Fetal magnetic resonance imaging of the central nervous system: a pictorial essay. *Eur Radiol* 2002;12:1952–61

24. Ertl-Wagner B, Lienemann A, Strauss A, *et al.* Fetal magnetic resonance imaging: indications, technique, anatomical considerations and a review of fetal abnormalities. *Eur Radiol* 2002;12:1931–40

25. Kubik-Huch RA, Huisman TA, Wisser J, *et al.* Ultrafast MR imaging of the fetus. *AJR* 2000;174:1599–606

26. Levine D, Barnes PD. Cortical maturation in normal and abnormal fetuses as assessed with prenatal MR imaging. *Radiology* 1999;210:751–8

27. Huppert BJ, Brandt KR, Ramin KD, *et al.* Single-shot fast spin-echo MR imaging of the fetus: a pictorial essay. *Radiographics* 1999;19:S215–27

28. Amin RS, Nikolaidis P, Kawashima A, *et al.* Normal anatomy of the fetus at MR imaging. *Radiographics* 1999;19:S201–14

4

Imaging of the normal fetal central nervous system

R.K. Pooh

CRANIAL BONE

The calvaria and its major sutures develop between 12 and 18 weeks of fetal life, with dura as guiding tissue in the morphogenesis of the skull[1]. The cranial bones are detectable by sonography from 10 weeks of gestation onwards. Figure 4.1 and 4.2 demonstrate the early fetal skull structure by two- and three-dimensional ultrasound. At 12 weeks, premature cranial bones and the sutures in between are detectable. The sagittal suture, lamboid sutures and posterior fontanelle are recognizable from 13 weeks. The diamond-shaped anterior fontanelle can be demonstrated after 15 weeks of gestation. As the fetal parietal portion has the anterior/posterior fontanelles and sagittal suture which is the widest suture among the fetal cranial sutures (Figure 4.3)[2], the transvaginal approach to the fetal brain using these spaces as ultrasound windows, demonstrates the detailed brain structure without the obstacle of the cranial bone, and is the most effective way for brain assessment.

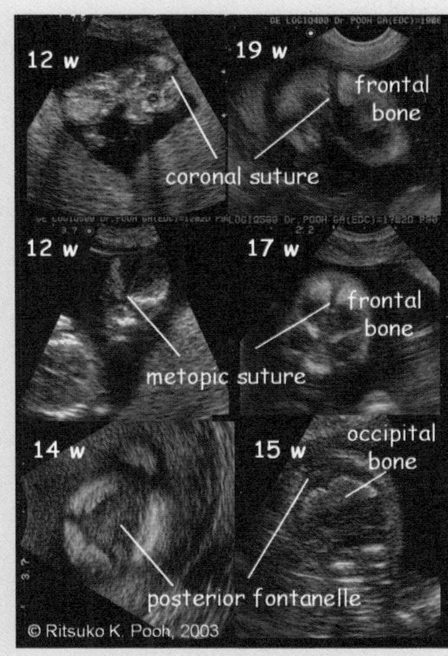

Figure 4.1 The fetal skull in early pregnancy. Two-dimensional ultrasound can demonstrate the fetal skull formation from an early stage. The most remarkable morphological change during early pregnancy is the metopic suture change. The V-shaped metopic suture between the bilateral frontal bones at 12 weeks changes into a linear structure at around 17 weeks

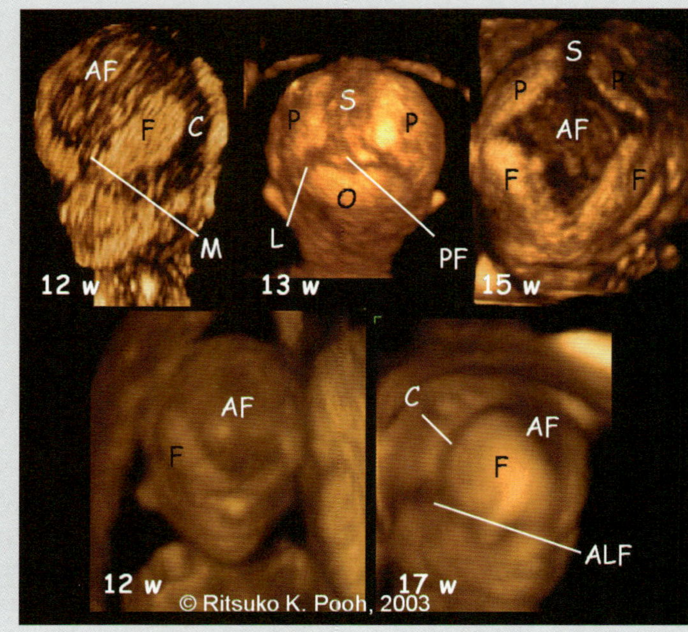

Figure 4.2 The fetal cranial structure in early gestation (three-dimensional ultrasound images). Upper left, 12 weeks, from the oblique front. Upper middle, 13 weeks, from the back. Upper right, 15 weeks, from the top of the head. Lower left, 12 weeks, from the front. Lower right, 17 weeks, oblique position. The premature shapes of the cranial bones, sutures and fontanelles at 12–13 weeks gradually change their appearance to the neonatal cranial shape. AF, anterior fontanelle; PF, posterior fontanelle; ALF, anterolateral fontanelle; F, frontal bone; P, parietal bone; O, occipital bone; C, coronal suture; M, metopic suture; S, sagittal suture; L, lamboid suture

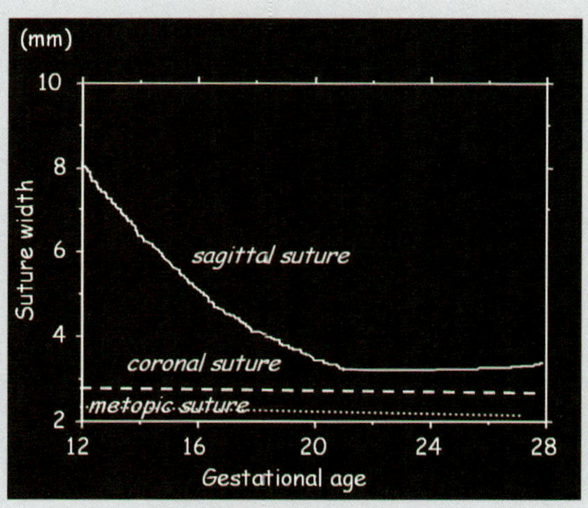

Figure 4.3 Suture width change during normal pregnancy. The change of suture width between 12 and 28 weeks of gestation. Sagittal suture is the widest suture. This fact indicates that transvaginal sonography is a reasonable way to approach the fetal brain

INTRACRANIAL STRUCTURE

As described in Chapter 2, the brain should be understood as a three-dimensional structure. Figures 4.4–4.9 show normal fetal brain images in the same cutting section at different gestational ages. By use of transvaginal three-dimensional sonography as described in Chapter 3, serial tomographic images in the three orthogonal sections can be demonstrated. Figures 4.10–4.17 show serial parallel sectional images of normal fetuses in the sagittal, coronal and axial planes at 8, 11, 15, 19, 24, 27, 31 and 36 weeks of gestation. Gyral formation is observed from approximately 26–28 weeks of gestation by

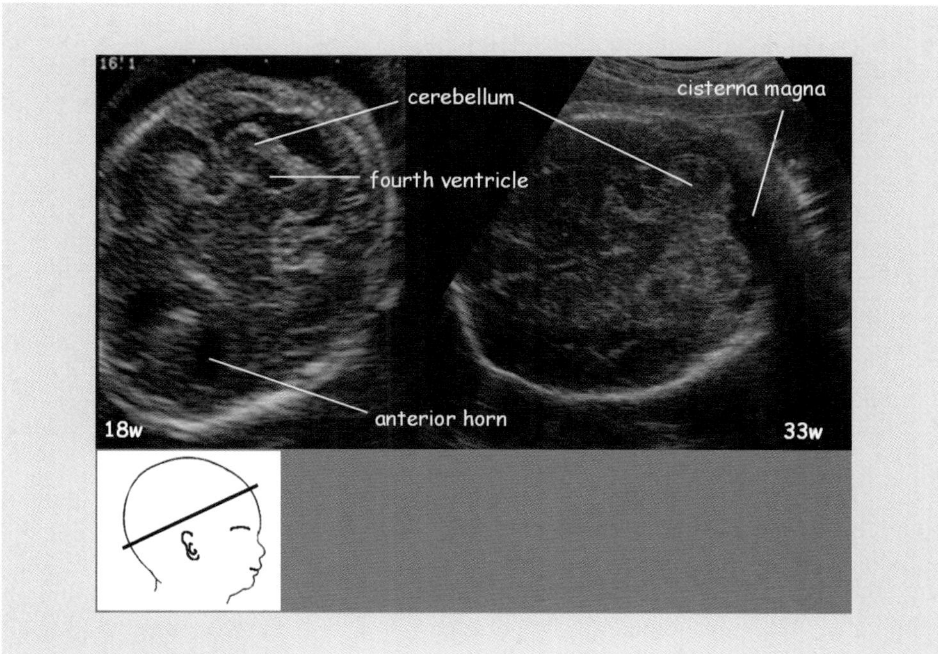

Figure 4.4 Axial sections at 18 and 33 weeks of gestation

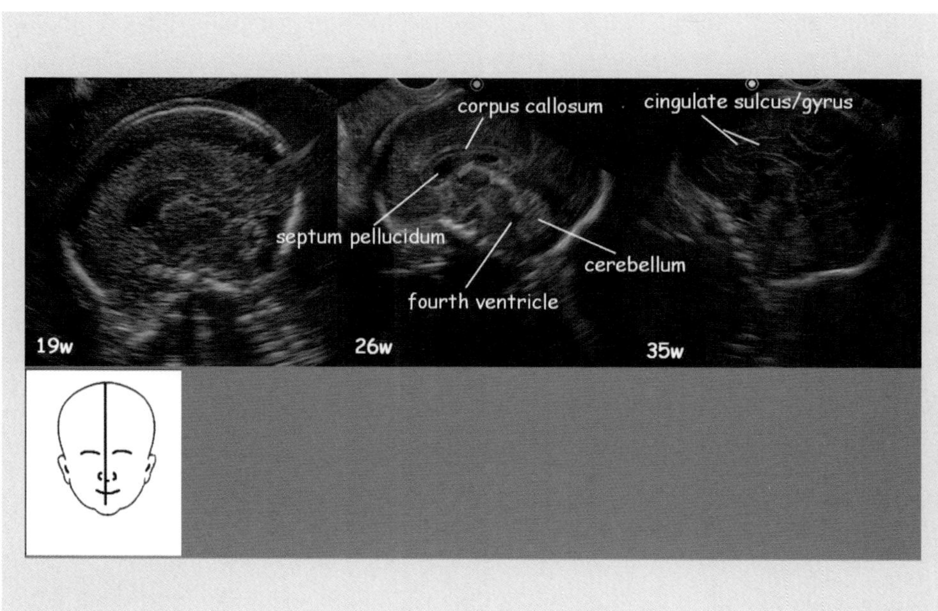

Figure 4.5 Sagittal sections at 19, 26 and 35 weeks of gestation

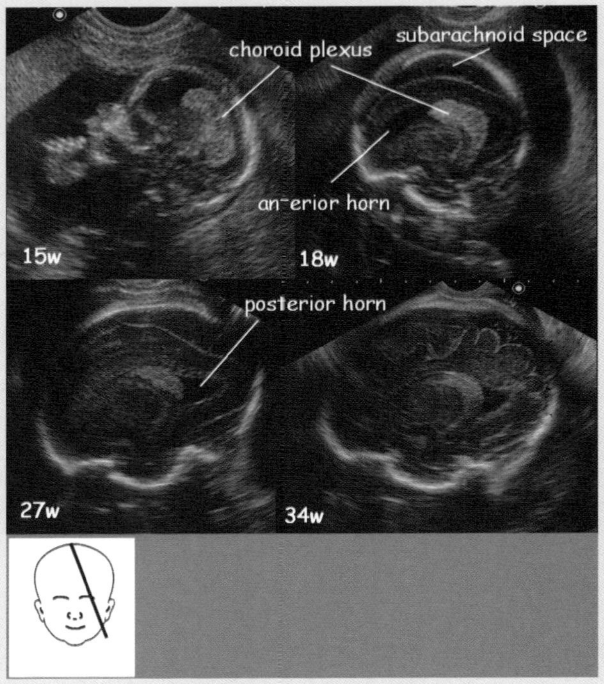

Figure 4.6 Parasagittal sections at 15, 18, 27 and 34 weeks of gestation

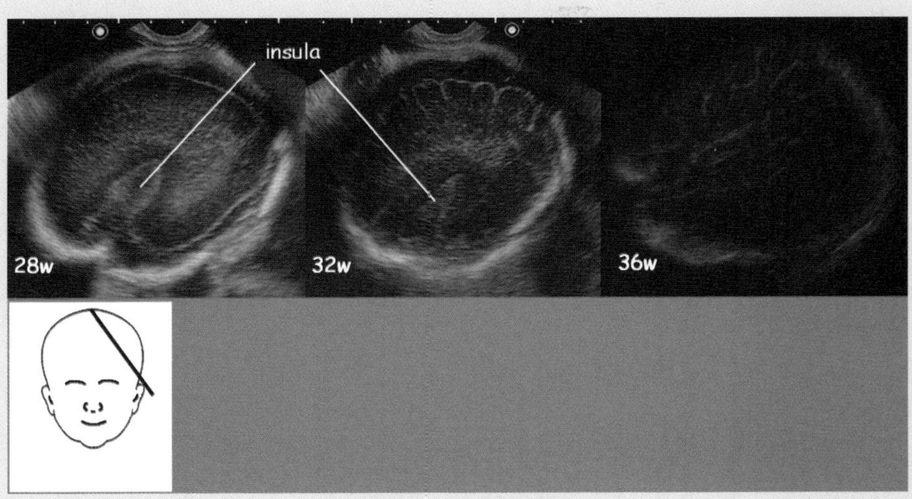

Figure 4.7 Parasagittal sections at 28, 32 and 36 weeks of gestation

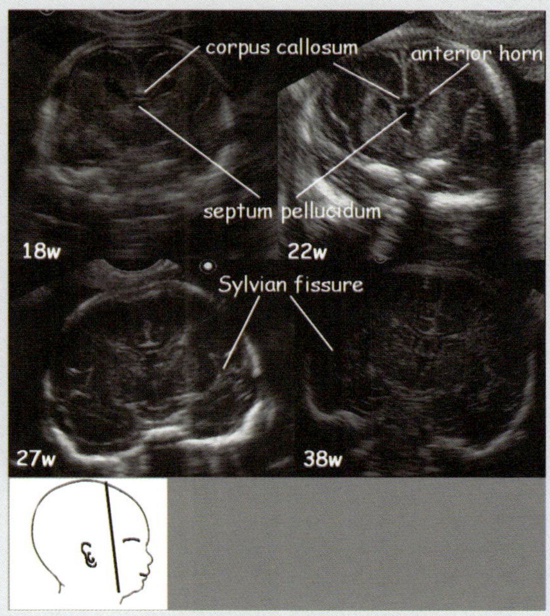

Figure 4.8 Anterior coronal sections at 18, 22, 27 and 38 weeks of gestation

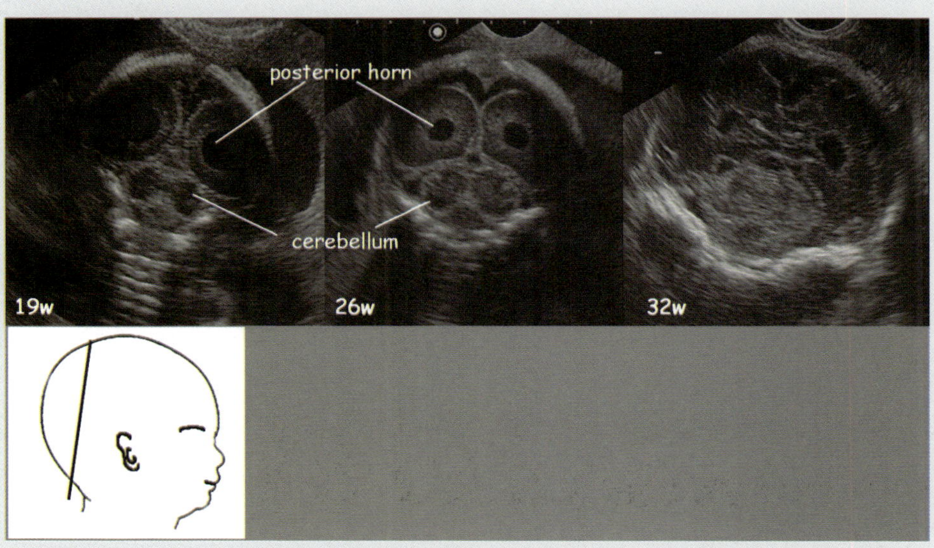

Figure 4.9 Posterior coronal sections at 19, 26 and 32 weeks of gestation

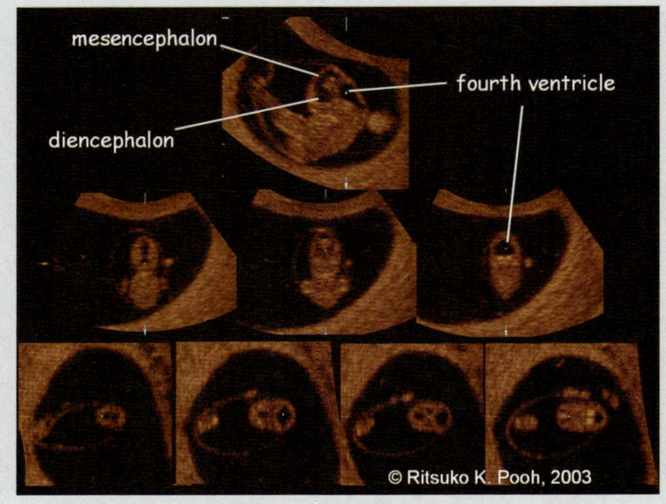

Figure 4.10 Normal intracranial structure at 8 weeks of gestation in parallel cutting slices of three orthogonal views; sagittal, coronal and axial sections from above. The premature sonolucent ventricular system is visible

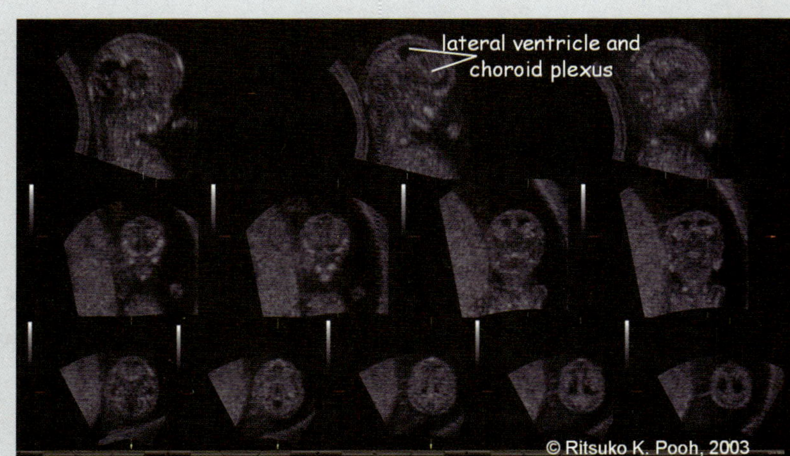

Figure 4.11 Normal intracranial structure at 11 weeks of gestation in parallel cutting slices of three orthogonal views; sagittal, coronal and axial sections from above

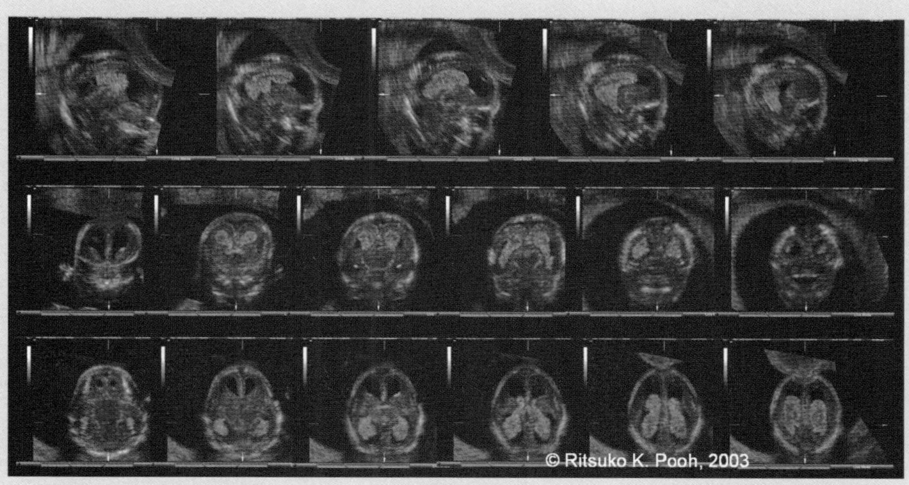

Figure 4.12 Normal intracranial structure at 15 weeks of gestation in parallel cutting slices of three orthogonal views; sagittal, coronal and axial sections from above

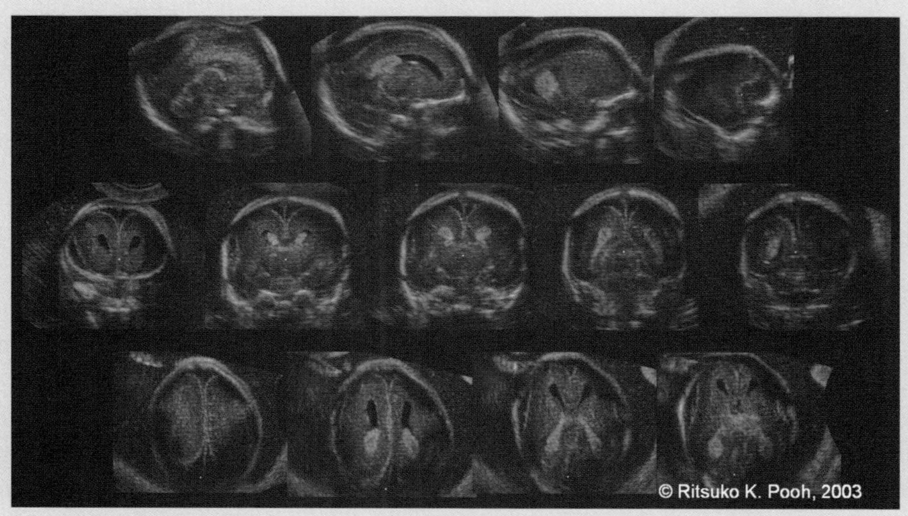

Figure 4.13 Normal intracranial structure at 19 weeks of gestation in parallel cutting slices of three orthogonal views; sagittal, coronal and axial sections from above

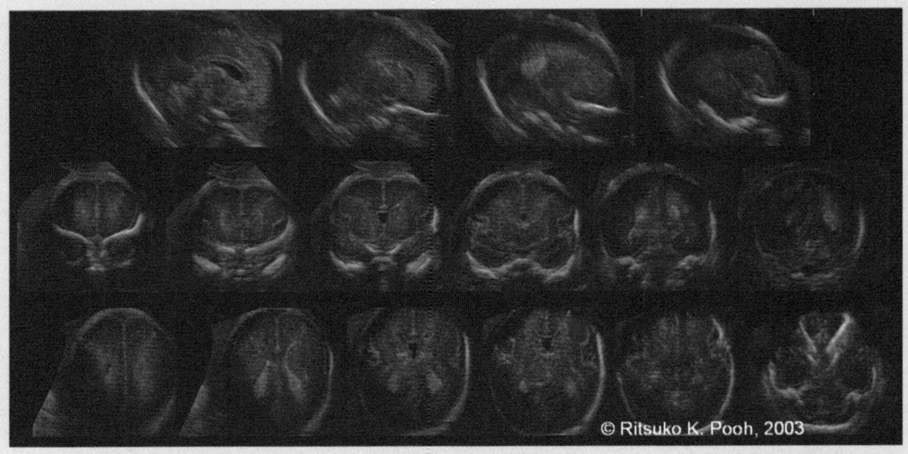

Figure 4.14 Normal intracranial structure at 24 weeks of gestation in parallel cutting slices of three orthogonal views; sagittal, coronal and axial sections from above

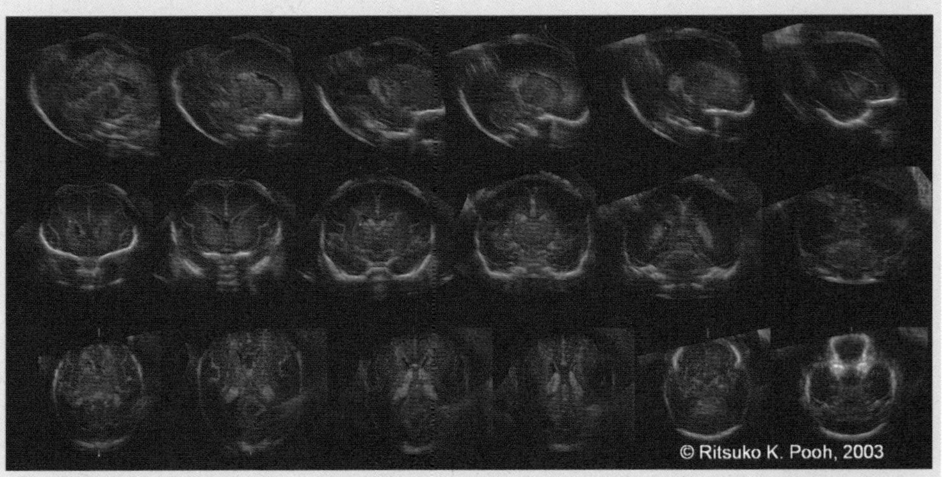

Figure 4.15 Normal intracranial structure at 27 weeks of gestation in parallel cutting slices of three orthogonal views; sagittal, coronal and axial sections from above

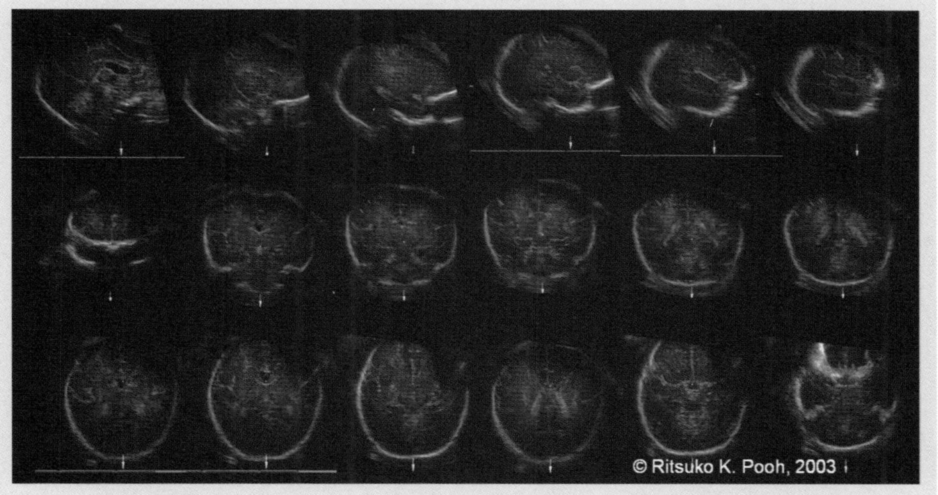

Figure 4.16 Normal intracranial structure at 31 weeks of gestation in parallel cutting slices of three orthogonal views; sagittal, coronal and axial sections from above

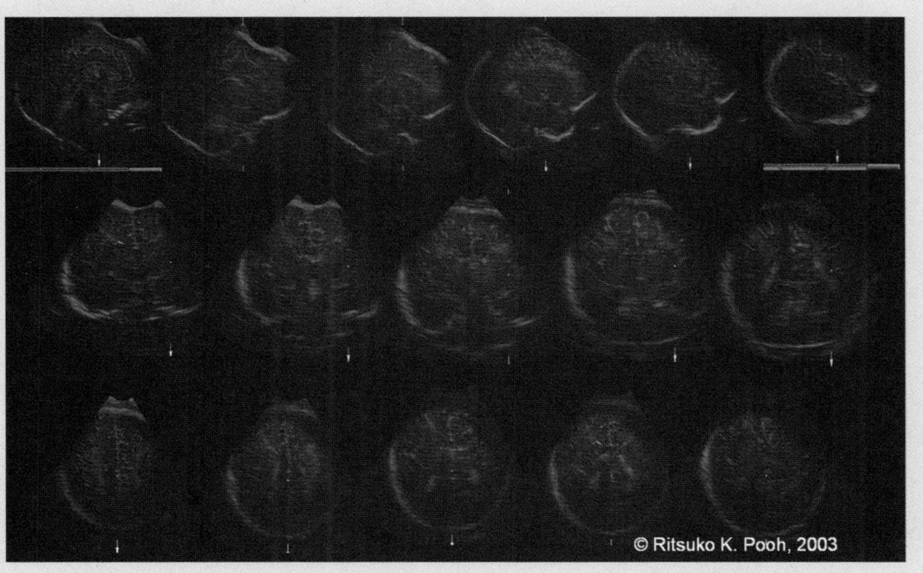

Figure 4.17 Normal intracranial structure at 36 weeks of gestation in parallel cutting slices of three orthogonal views; sagittal, coronal and axial sections from above. Note the gyral formation in the late pregnancy

sonography. After 30 weeks, sulci and gyri are well demonstrated as shown in Figure 4.18. Isolated lateral ventricular asymmetry is often detected as the area difference between the left and right ventricles in fetuses during the latter half of pregnancy (Figure 4.19) or in neonates. In most cases, an asymmetry resolves spontaneously during pregnancy or after birth and generally has no clinical significance and may be a normal variation. Ventricular asymmetry should be differentiated from the initial sign of progressive unilateral hydrocephalus or a rare developmental malformation such as unilateral megalencephaly.

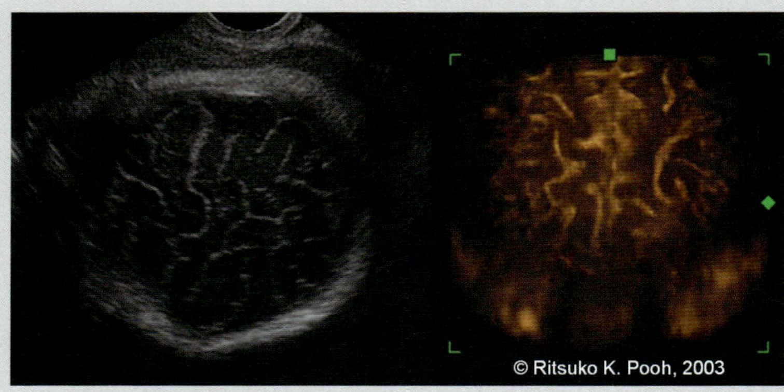

Figure 4.18 Gyral formation in the late pregnancy by two-dimensional (left) and three-dimensional (right) ultrasound

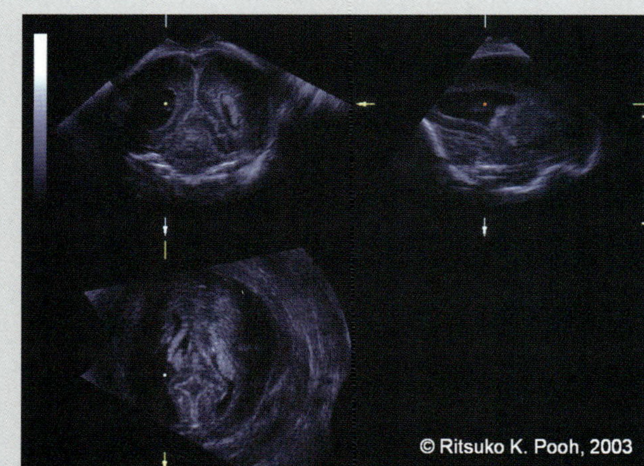

Figure 4.19 Lateral ventricular asymmetry (normal variation). Asymmetry of lateral ventricles are often observed in normal fetuses

VERTEBRAE AND SPINE

Vertebrae and spine should be observed carefully for the detection of back abnormalities such as spina bifida or scoliosis. The fetal sagittal sectional screening method is preferable (Figures 4.20 and 4.21). Three-dimensional ultrasound demonstrates the bony structure as shown in Figure 4.22 and recent advanced three-dimensional ultrasound has been able to depict vertebral body, intervertebral disk space and vertebral lamina (Figure 4.23).

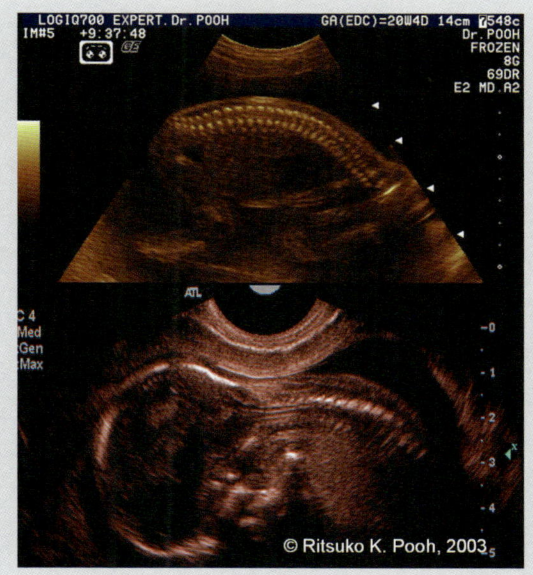

Figure 4.20 Vertebrae and spine in the sagittal section at 20 weeks of gestation

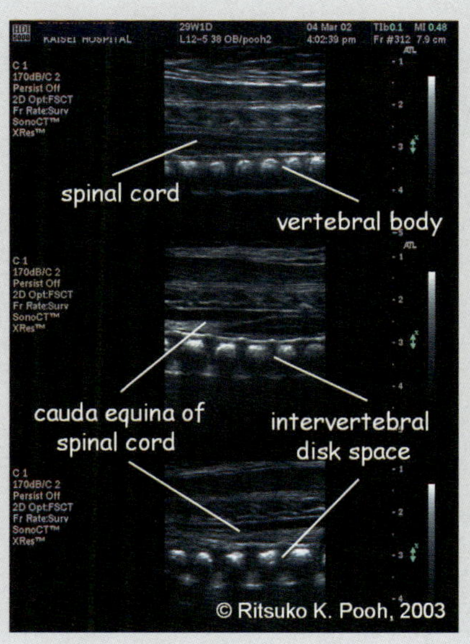

Figure 4.21 Vertebrae and spine in the sagittal section at 29 weeks of gestation. Upper, thoracic vertebrae; middle, lumbar vertebrae; lower, lumbosacral vertebrae

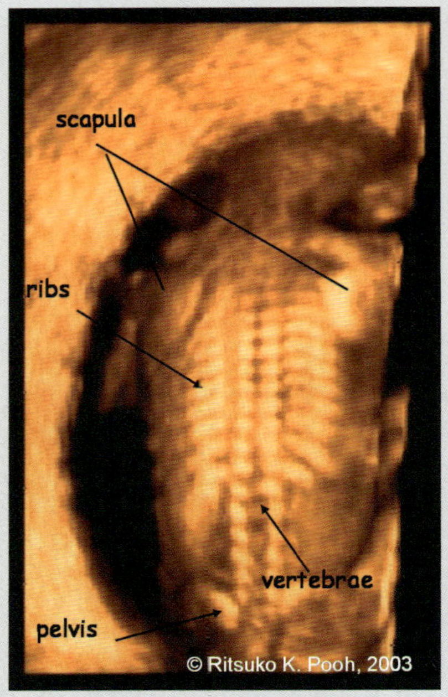

Figure 4.22 Fetal bony structure at 17 weeks of gestation

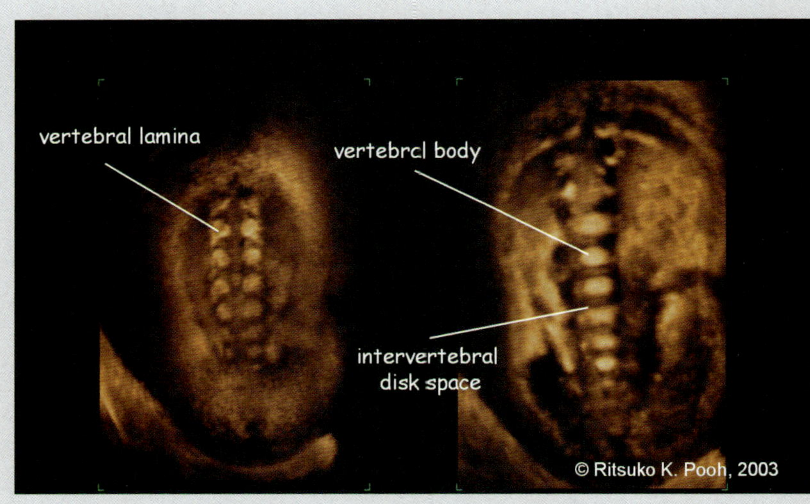

Figure 4.23 Fetal vertebral structure by three-dimensional ultrasound at 21 weeks of gestation

BRAIN CIRCULATION

Intracranial blood vessels can be visualized by color/power Doppler from early pregnancy (Figure 4.24). Transvaginal power Doppler demonstrates clear anatomical vascular formation (Figure 4.25). Dural sinuses such as the superior sagittal sinus, vein of Galen and straight sinus are located in the median section. Therefore, the transvaginal sagittal view demonstrates these dural sinuses (Figure 4.26). In normal cases, venous blood flow waveforms have pulsations as shown in Figure 4.26, while in cases with progressive hydrocephalus, the pulsatile pattern disappears (see Chapter 5). Intracranial circulatory structure can be well demonstrated by three-dimensional power Doppler[3] (Figure 4.27).

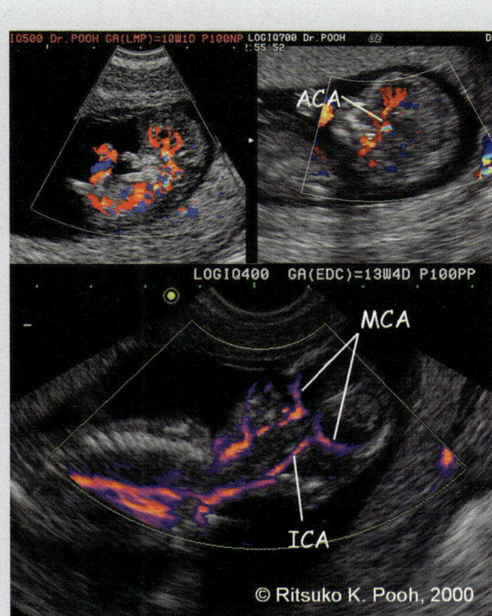

Figure 4.24 Intercerebral circulation by color/power Doppler in early pregnancy. Upper left, sagittal image at 10 weeks of gestation. Premature arterial vessels toward the brain are visualized. Upper right, sagittal image at 12 weeks. Branches of the anterior cerebral artery (ACA) are demonstrated. Lower, coronal image at 13 weeks. Bilateral internal carotid arteries (ICA) and middle cerebral arteries (MCA) are demonstrated

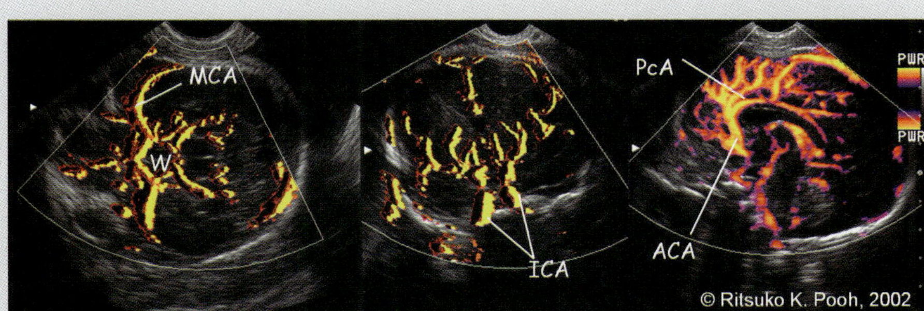

Figure 4.25 Brain circulation by two-dimensional power Doppler. Left, axial image. Circle of Willis (W) and middle cerebral arteries (MCA) are demonstrated. Middle, coronal image. Internal carotid arteries (ICA) and branches of the middle cerebral arteries are visible. Right, sagittal image. Anterior cerebral artery (ACA), pericallosal artery (PcA) and branches are demonstrated

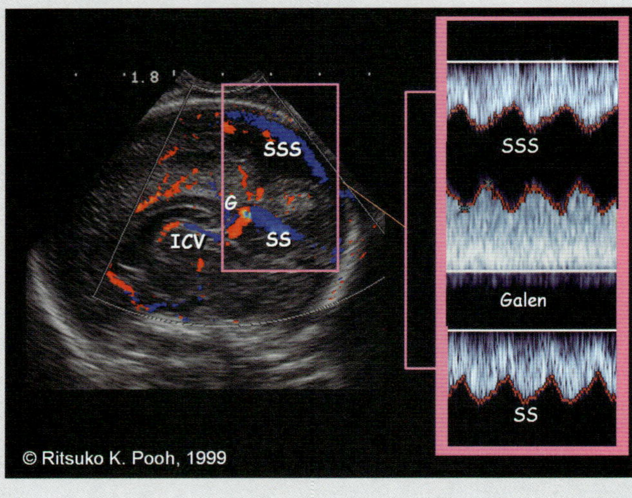

Figure 4.26 Normal cerebral venous circulation. Left, sagittal image of color Doppler. SSS, superior, sagittal sinus; ICV, internal cerebral vein; G, vein of Galen; SS, straight sinus. Right, normal blood flow waveforms of dural sinuses. In normal fetuses, venous flow always has pulsations

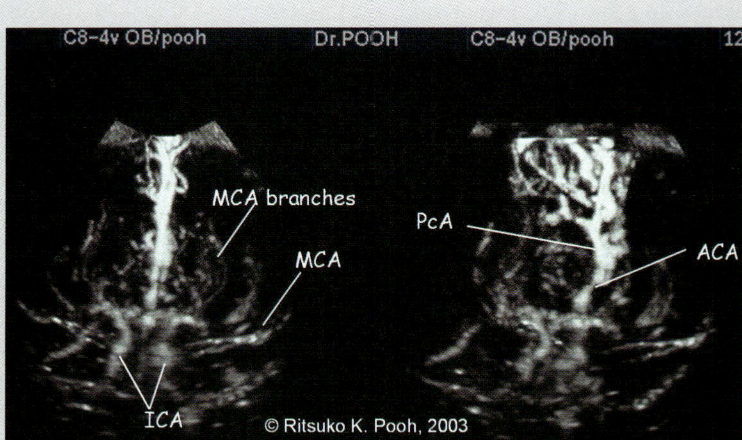

Figure 4.27 Three-dimensional power Doppler image of fetal brain circulation. Left, view from the front. Bilateral internal carotid arteries (ICA) and middle cerebral arteries (MCA) and branches of MCA are demonstrated. Right, oblique view. Anterior cerebral artery (ACA) and pericallosal artery (PcA) are demonstrated

VOLUME CALCULATION

Volume analysis by three-dimensional ultrasound provides exceedingly informative imaging data. Volume analysis of the structure of interest provides an intelligible evaluation of the brain structure in total, and longitudinal and objective assessment of enlarged ventricles and intracranial occupying lesions. Any intracranial organ can be chosen as a target for volumetry no matter how distorted its shape and appearance may be[4,5]. Figures 4.28–4.30 show the volume measurement of the intracranial cavity, the lateral ventricle and the choroid plexus in normal fetuses and their normal development during pregnancy. Figure 4.31 shows the changing appearance of the lateral ventricle and choroid plexus during pregnancy.

VOLUME CONTRAST IMAGES BY FOUR-DIMENSIONAL TECHNOLOGY

Recent advances in three- and four-dimensional ultrasound technology has enabled us to demonstrate the thick-slice images, which have been utilized in MRI technology. Using this technology of volume contrast imaging, real-time images with increased contrast resolution can be obtained as described in Chapter 3. Figure 4.32 shows a volume contrast image of cerebral sulci at 33 weeks. It is possible to demonstrate the thick-slice vertical to a two-dimensional image by the same technology (Figures 4.33 and 4.34). The novel unique technology of volume contrast imaging provides additional information simultaneously with conventional two-dimensional imaging, without the process of off-line three-dimensional reconstruction[6].

MAGNETIC RESONANCE IMAGING

Recent advances in fast MRI technology have produced high-resolution images without fetal sedation or fetal/maternal motion artifact despite a short acquisition time. MRI demonstrates the brain structure in detail (Figure 4.35), including the brainstem which cannot be clearly depicted even by transvaginal sonography. Surface anatomical MRI demonstrates the outer surface of the brain. Figure 4.36 shows the surface gyral formation of the cerebrum.

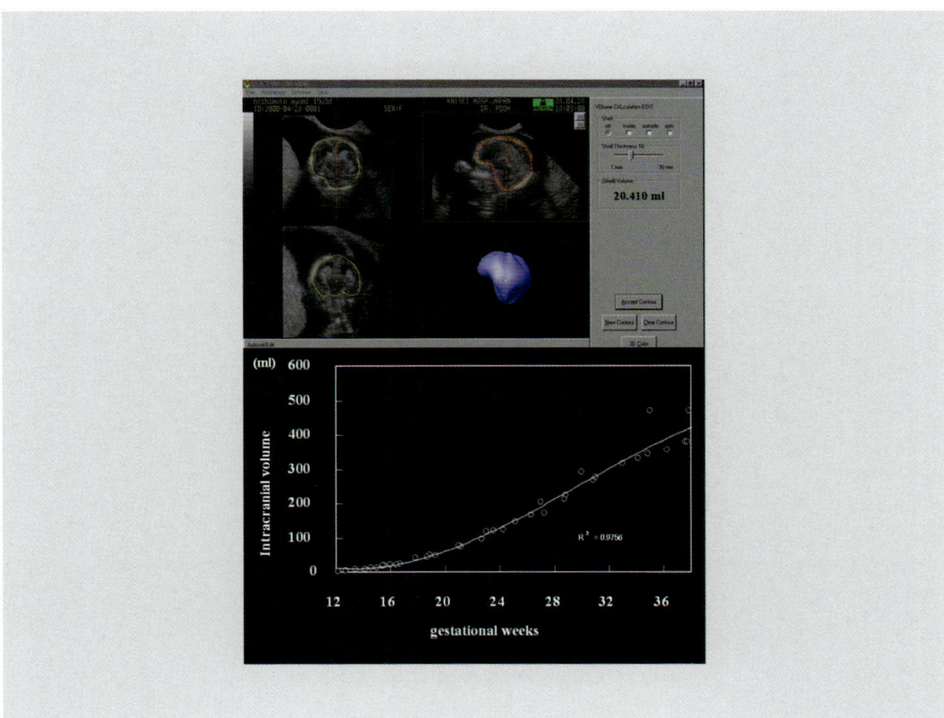

Figure 4.28 Intracranial cavity volume during pregnancy. Upper, three orthogonal views and volume extraction image of a 15-week-old fetus. Lower, nomogram of intracranial volume during pregnancy

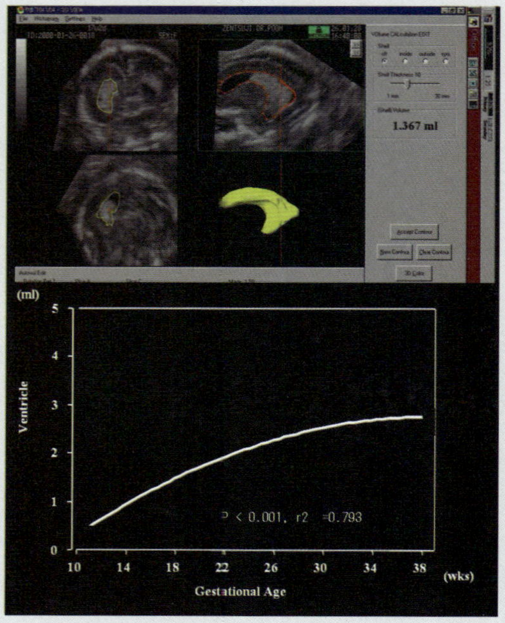

Figure 4.29 Lateral ventricular volume during pregnancy. Upper, three orthogonal views and volume extraction image of a 17-week-old fetus. Lower, nomogram of lateral ventricular volume during pregnancy

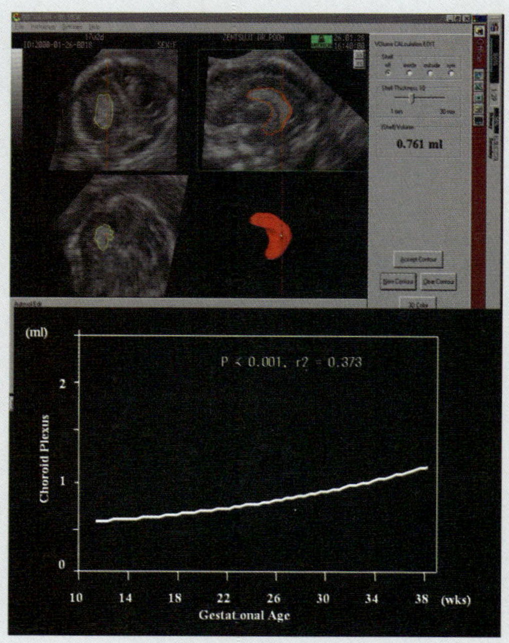

Figure 4.30 Choroid plexus volume during pregnancy. Upper, three orthogonal views and volume extraction image of a 17-week-old fetus. Lower, nomogram of choroid plexus volume during pregnancy

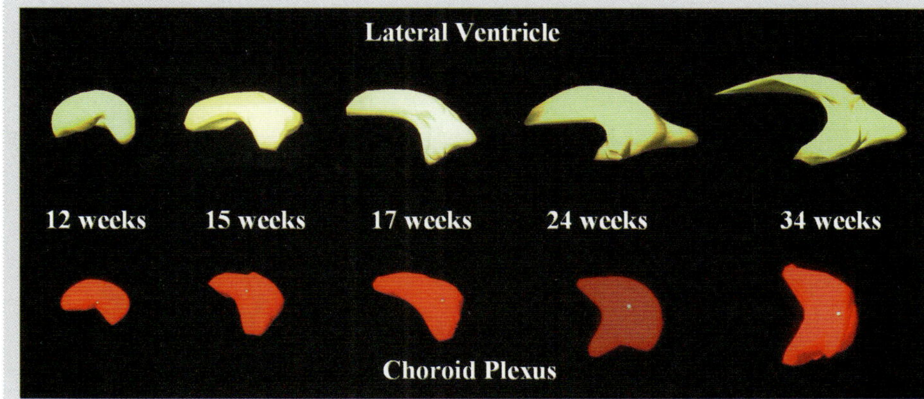

Figure 4.31 Changing appearance of the lateral ventricle and choroid plexus between 12 and 34 weeks (three-dimensional ultrasound volume extraction image). Upper, lateral ventricle; lower, choroid plexus

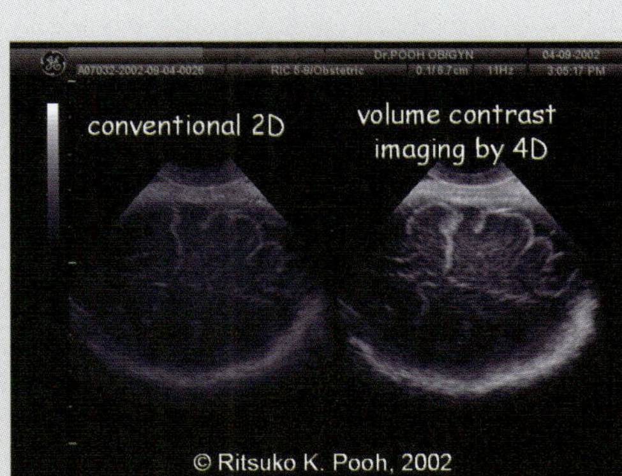

Figure 4.32 Simultaneous volume contrast imaging by four-dimensional technology. Cerebral gyral formation at 33 weeks of gestation. Conventional two-dimensional imaging and volume contrast imaging, which means a thick slice image, are simultaneously demonstrated

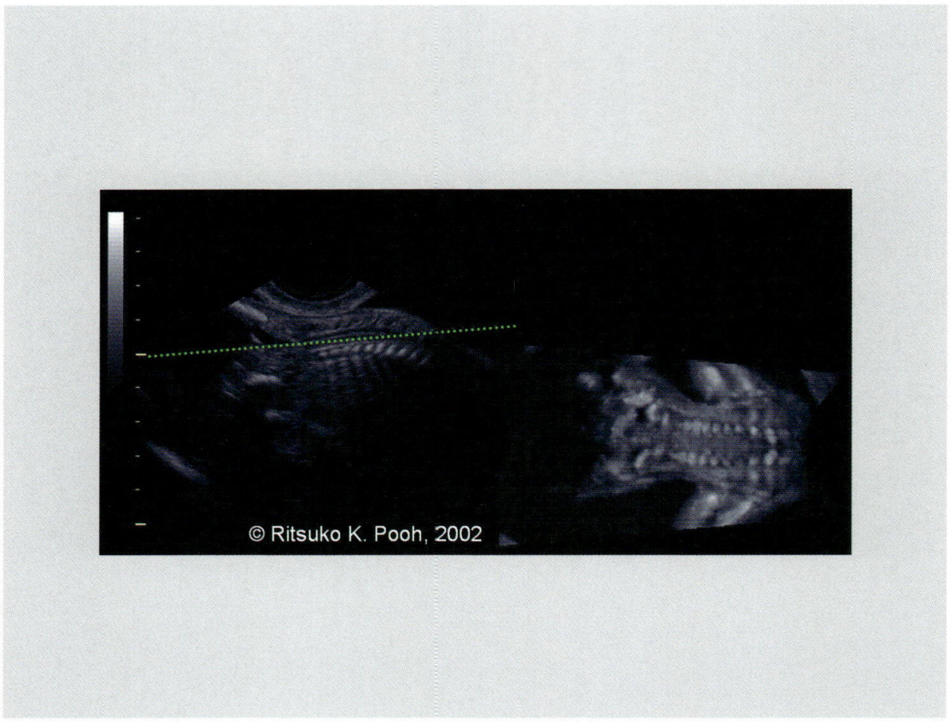

Figure 4.33 Simultaneous volume contrast imaging of the vertical plane by four-dimensional technology. Fetal spinal cord and vertebrae at 19 weeks of gestation. Left, conventional two-dimensional image. Right, thick slice of the vertical section plane of a two-dimensional image is simultaneously demonstrated

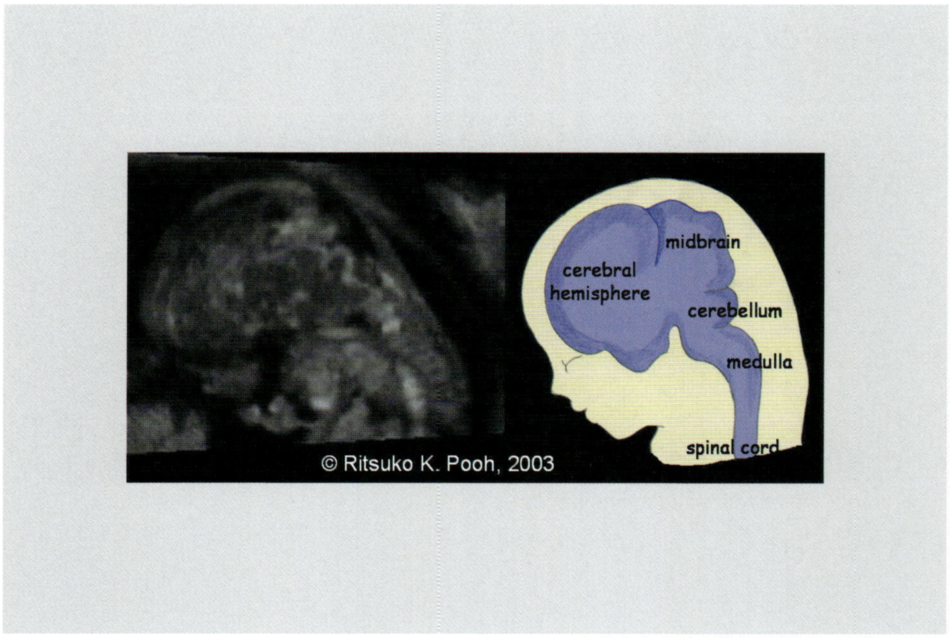

Figure 4.34 Simultaneous volume contrast imaging of the vertical plane by four-dimensional technology. Developing midbrain, cerebellum and medulla at 14 weeks of gestation. Left, volume contrast image; right, schema indicates the development of the premature brain at the same gestation

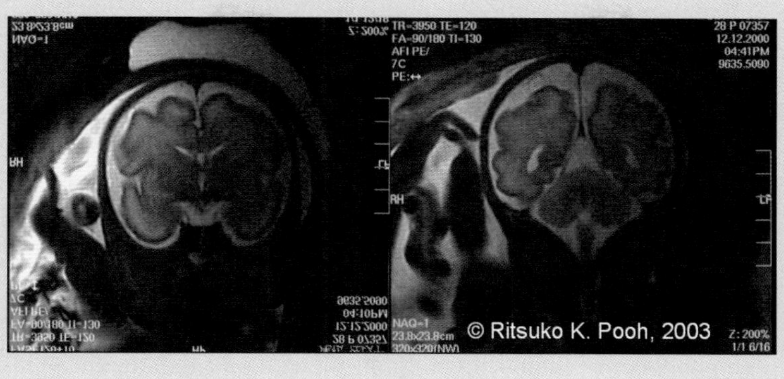

Figure 4.35 Magnetic resonance coronal images of a normal fetal brain at 33 weeks of gestation. Left, anterior coronal image; right, posterior coronal image. Note the subarachnoid space around the cerebral surface

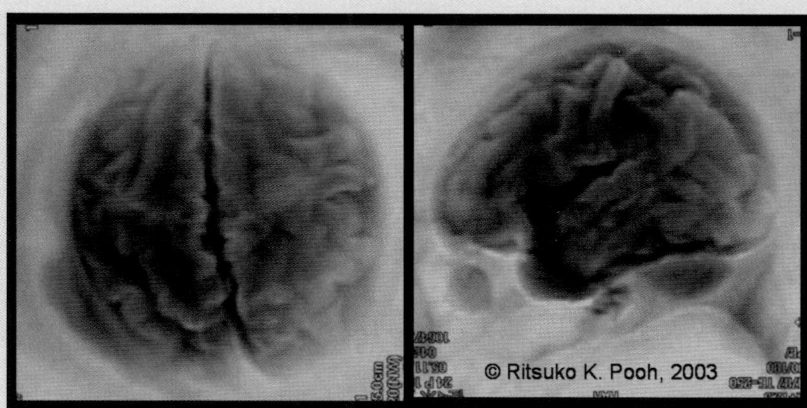

Figure 4.36 Magnetic resonance surface anatomical imaging of a fetal brain at 34 weeks of gestation. Left, bilateral hemispheres; right, lateral view of left hemisphere

REFERENCES

1. Smith DW, Tondury G. Origin of the calvaria and its sutures. *Am J Dis Child* 1978;132:662–6
2. Pooh RK. Fetal cranial bone formation: sonographic assessment. In Margulies M, Voto LS, Eik-Nes S, eds. *9th World Congress of Ultrasound in Obstetrics and Gynecology*. Bologna, Italy: Monduzzi Editore, 1999:407–10
3. Pooh RK, Pooh KH. The assessment of fetal brain morphology and circulation by transvaginal 3D sonography and power Doppler. *J Perinat Med* 2002;30:48–56
4. Pooh RK, Pooh KH. Transvaginal 3D and Doppler ultrasonography of the fetal brain. *Semin Perinatol* 2001;25:38–43
5. Pooh RK, Pooh KH. Transvaginal three-dimensional volume assessment of the fetal brain structure. In Chervenak FA, Kurjak A, Papp Z, eds. *The Fetus as a Patient, The Evolving Challenge*. London: Parthenon Publishing, 2002:73–7
6. Pooh RK, Pooh KH. Fetal neuroimaging with new technology. *Ultrasound Rev Obstet Gynecol* 2002;2:178–81

5

Hydrocephalus and ventriculomegaly

R.K. Pooh and K.H. Pooh

PRENATAL ASSESSMENT OF ENLARGED VENTRICLES

Hydrocephalus and ventriculomegaly *in utero*

The two terms, hydrocephalus and ventriculomegaly, are often used to describe dilatation of the lateral ventricles. However, they should be distinguished from each other in order to assess the enlargement of the ventricles. Hydrocephalus is a dilatation of the lateral ventricles resulting from an increased amount of cerebrospinal fluid (CSF) and increased intracranial pressure, while ventriculomegaly is a dilatation of the lateral ventricles without increased intracranial pressure due to hypoplastic cerebrum or other intracerebral abnormalities such as agenesis of the corpus callosum. Of course, ventriculomegaly can sometimes change into the hydrocephalic state. In sonographic imaging, these two intracranial conditions can be differentiated by visualization of the subarachnoid space and the appearance of the choroid plexus. In normal conditions, the subarachnoid space, visualized around both cerebral hemispheres (Figures 5.1 and 5.2), is preserved during pregnancy. The choroid plexus, which secretes CSF within the ventricles, is a soft tissue and is easily affected by pressure (Figure 5.2). The transvaginal coronal and parasagittal (oblique) images demon-

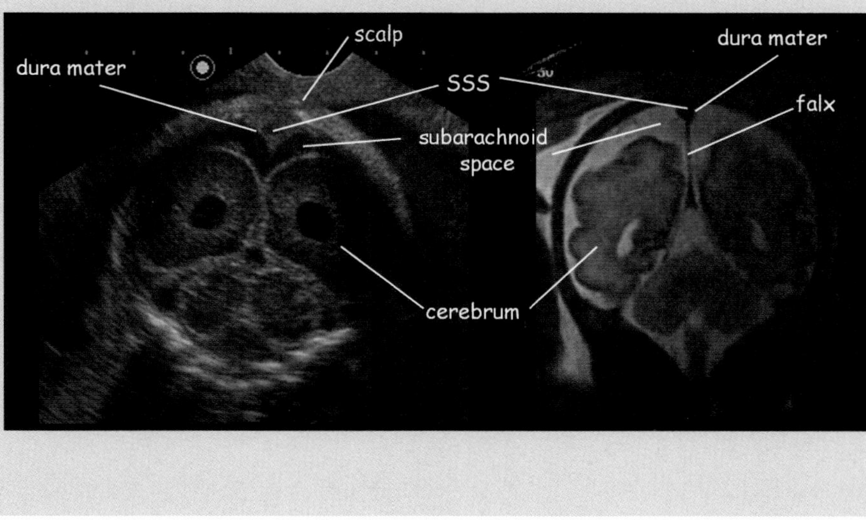

Figure 5.1 Normal structure outside the cerebral hemispheres. Outside the hemispheres, the subarachnoid space is normally observed. Outside the subarachnoid space, dura mater, cranial bone and the scalp cover the brain. SSS, superior sagittal sinus

strate the obliterated subarachnoid space and the dangling choroid plexus in the case of hydrocephalus (Figure 5.3). In contrast, the subarachnoid space and choroid plexus are well preserved in cases of ventriculomegaly[1] (Figure 5.4). It is difficult to evaluate obliterated subarachnoid space by the transabdominal approach which may not accurately differentiate hydrocephalus with increased intracranial pressure from ventriculomegaly without pressure. Therefore, it is suggested that the evaluation of fetuses with enlarged ventricles should be evaluated in the parasagittal and coronal views by the transvaginal way or three-dimensional multiplanar analysis. Figures 5.5–5.9 show sonographic images of hydrocephalus from early to late gestation. In early pregnancy, the subarachnoid space is not depicted even in normal fetuses. However, the choroid plexus is dangling and deviates toward the occipital portion

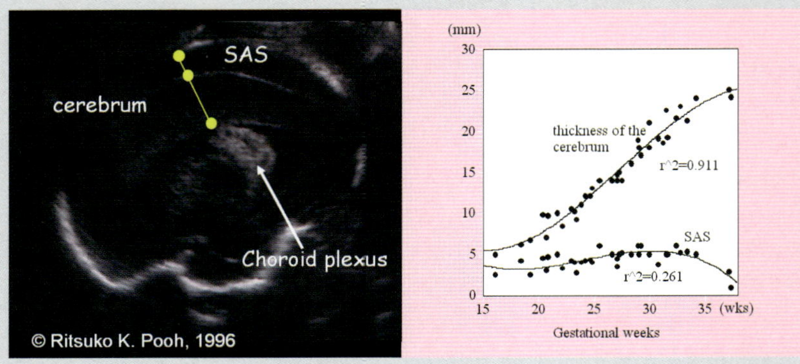

Figure 5.2 Subarachnoid space in a normal fetus. The subarachnoid space (SAS), which is demonstrated around the cerebral hemispheres is preserved during pregnancy. Right, graph shows the width change of subarachnoid space and the thickness of the cerebrum during a normal pregnancy

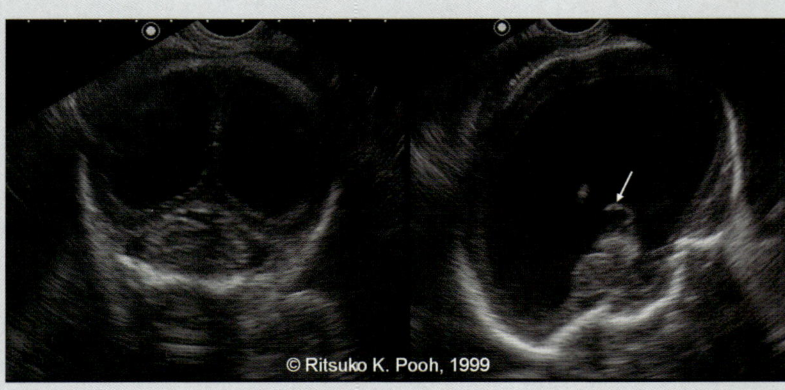

Figure 5.3 Ultrasound images of fetal hydrocephalus at 34 weeks of gestation. Left, coronal image. The subarachnoid space is obliterated. Right, sagittal image. A dangling choroid plexus is demonstrated (arrow)

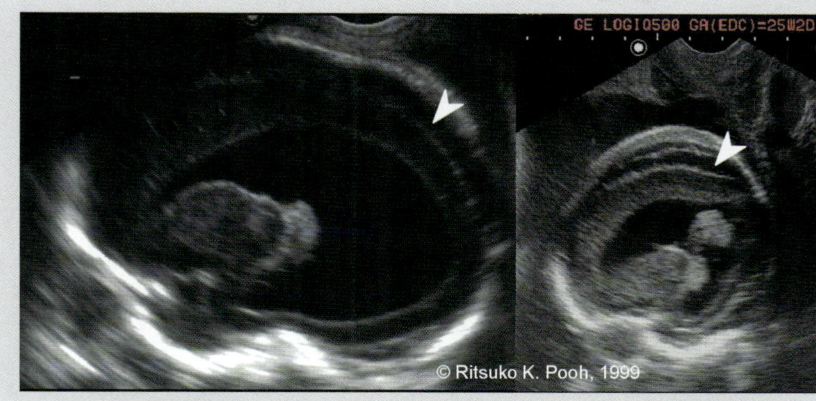

Figure 5.4 Ultrasound images of ventriculomegaly. Enlarged ventricles exist but the subarachnoid space (arrowheads) is well preserved and there is no dangling choroid plexus, which indicates normal intercranial pressure. This condition should be differentiated from hydrocephalus

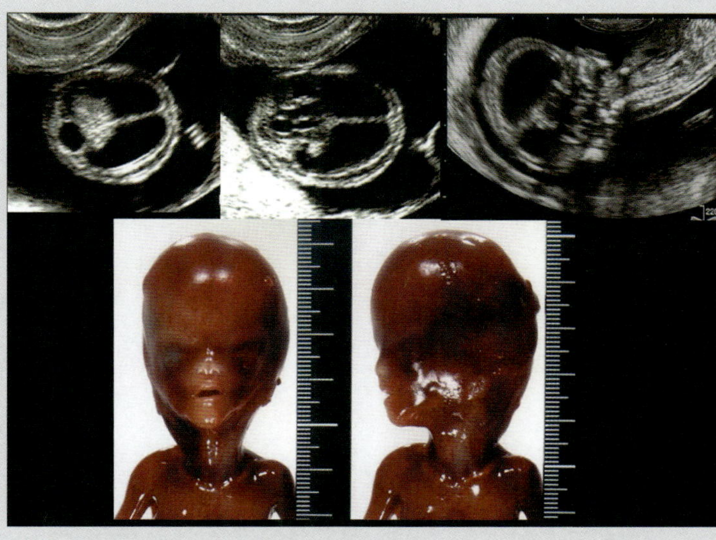

Figure 5.5 Early hydrocephalus at 10–12 weeks of gestation. Upper left and middle, axial images at 10 weeks. Choroid plexus is replaced backwards in the ventricles and marked intraventricular fluid collection is demonstrated. Upper right, sagittal image at 12 weeks. The fetal head is enlarged and frontal bossing is conspicuous. Lower, external appearance of the head and face in an aborted fetus at 14 weeks. Images and photographs courtesy of Dr T. Murakoshi

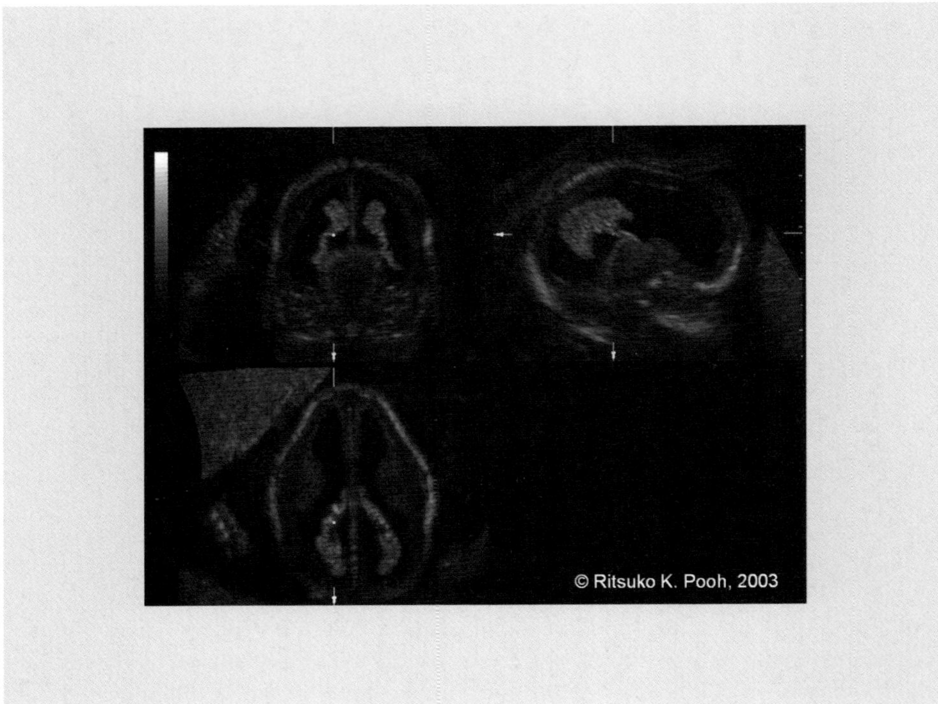

Figure 5.6 Three-dimensional orthogonal views of hydrocephalus at 16 weeks of gestation. Upper left, coronal image; upper right, sagittal image; lower, axial image. This case was complicated by myelomeningocele. The subarachnoid space is already obliterated and a dangling choroid plexus is seen

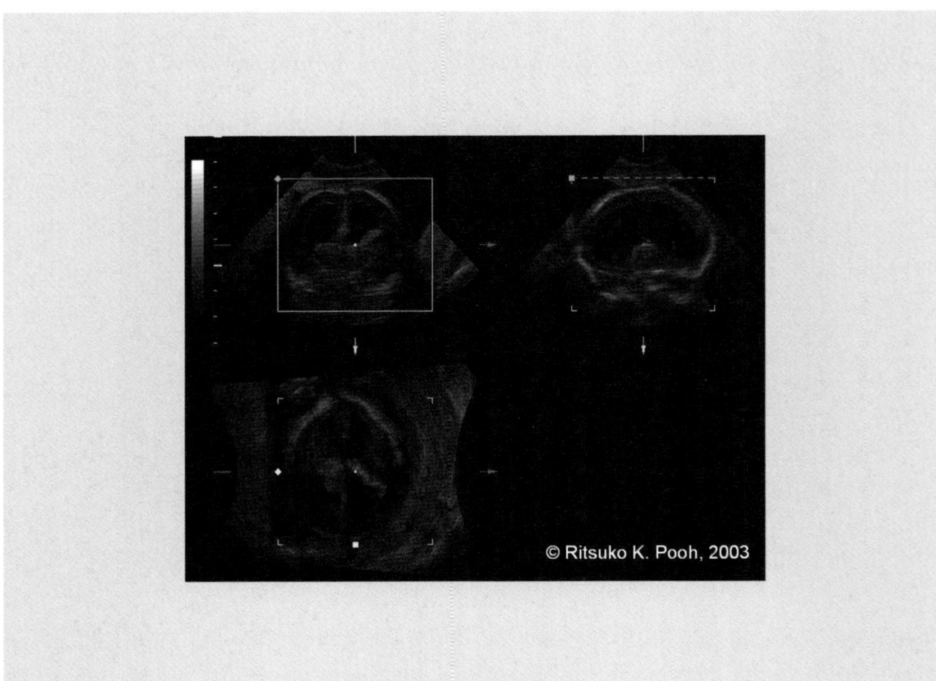

Figure 5.7 Three-dimensional orthogonal views of hydrocephalus at 18 weeks of gestation. Upper left, coronal image; upper right, sagittal image; lower, axial image. The subarachnoid space is already obliterated and a dangling choroid plexus is seen

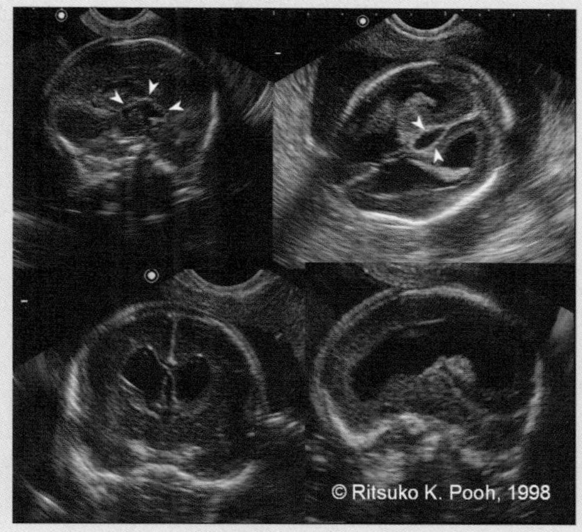

Figure 5.8 Hydrocephalus with third ventriculomegaly at 19 weeks of gestation. Upper left, sagittal ultrasound image; upper right, axial image. Mild enlargement of the third ventricle is demonstrated (arrowheads). Lower left, anterior coronal image of hydrocephalus. The septum pellucidum is intact. Lower right, parasagittal image. Note the obliterated subarachnoid space and dangling choroid plexus

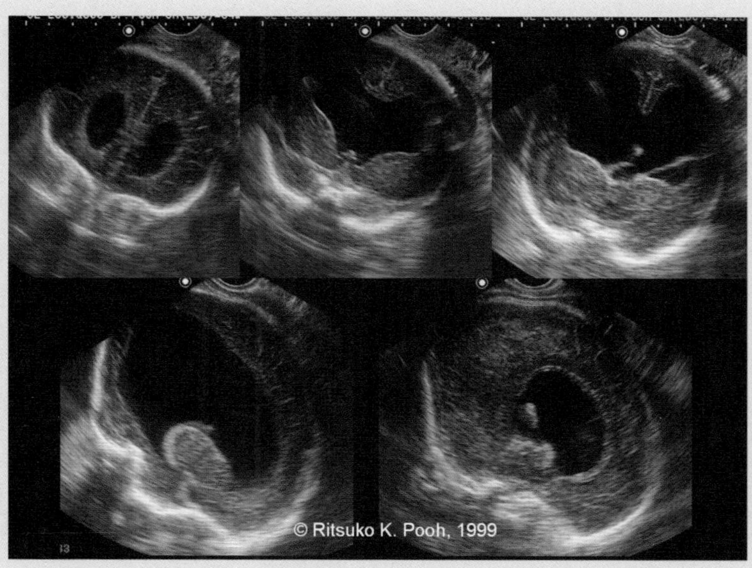

Figure 5.9 Ultrasound images of hydrocephalus at 34 weeks of gestation. Upper, serial coronal images. The septum pellucidum was destroyed, perhaps due to enlargement of the bilateral ventricles, and both ventricles were fused. A dangling choroid plexus is seen. Lower, parasagittal and sagittal images. A dangling choroid plexus and obliterated subarachnoid space are seen

of the lateral ventricles in a case of hydrocephalus as early as 10 weeks of gestation (Figure 5.5). Under normal conditions from the beginning of the second trimester, the subarachnoid space may be visible. The obliterated subarachnoid space and dangling choroid plexus are conspicuous (Figures 5.6–5.8). In some cases with hydrocephalus, the septum pellucidum is destroyed and both ventricles are fused together (Figure 5.9). This condition should be differentiated from the lobar type of holoprosencephaly. Furthermore, intracranial venous blood flow may be related to increased intracranial pressure. In normal fetuses, blood flow waveforms of dural sinuses, such as the superior sagittal sinus, vein of Galen and straight sinus have a pulsatile pattern[2] (see Chapter 4, Figure 4.26). However, in cases with progressive hydrocephalus, normal pulsation disappears and blood flow waveforms develop a flat pattern[2] (Figure 5.10). In cases with progressive hydrocephalus, there may be seven stages of progression (Figure 5.11):

(1) Increased fluid collection in the lateral ventricles;
(2) Increased intracranial pressure;
(3) Dangling choroid plexus;
(4) Disappearance of subarachnoid space;
(5) Excessive extension of the dura and superior sagittal sinus;
(6) Disappearance of venous pulsation;
(7) Enlarged skull.

In general, both hydrocephalus and ventriculomegaly are still evaluated by the measurement of biparietal diameter (BPD) and the lateral ventricular width/hemispheric width (LVW/HW) ratio in the transabdominal axial section. As described above, however, hydrocephalus and ventriculomegaly should be differentiated from each other and the hydrocephalic state should be assessed by the changing appearance of the intracranial structure. BPD and LVW/HW ratio may not exactly identify the intracranial condition. To evaluate enlarged ventricles, examiners should carefully observe the structures below and specify the causes of hydrocephalus:

- Choroid plexus, dangling or not
- Subarachnoid space, obliterated or not
- Ventricles, symmetry or asymmetry
- Visibility of third ventricle
- Pulsation of dural sinuses
- Ventricular size (three-dimensional volume calculation if possible)
- Other abnormalities

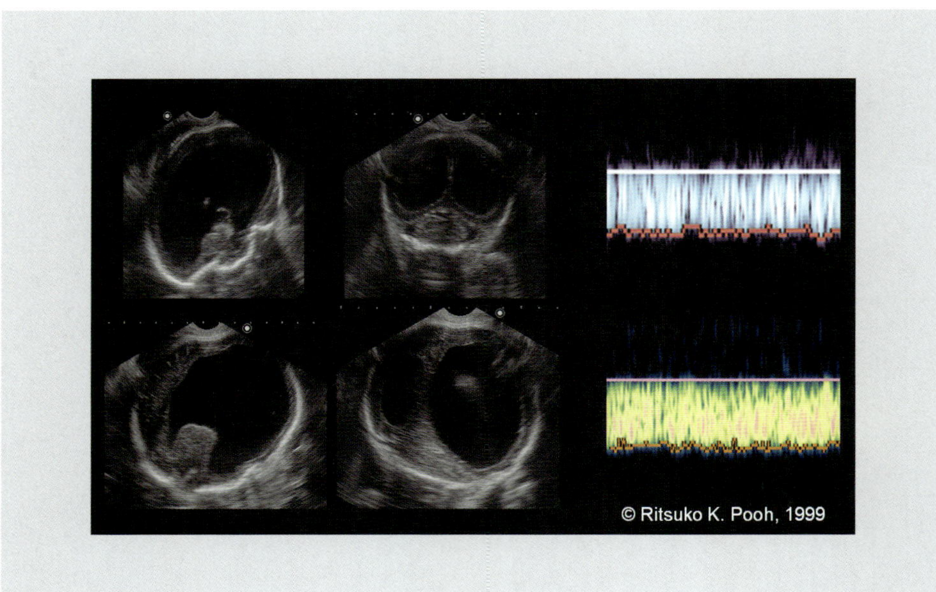

Figure 5.10 Disappearance of venous pulsation in cases with hydrocephalus. Normal dural sinuses have pulsatile patterns of flow waveform (Figure 4.26). In cases with progressive hydrocephalus, venous pulsation disappears (right) perhaps due to excessive extension of the dura and dural sinuses

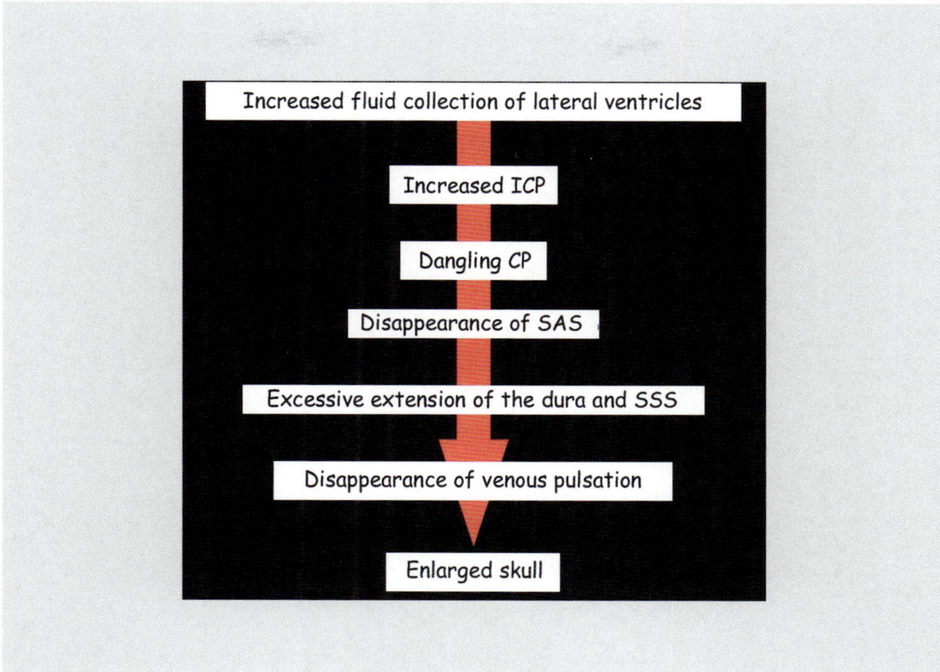

Figure 5.11 Progressive stages of hydrocephalus. ICP, intracranial pressure; CP, choroid plexus; SAS, subarachnoid space; SSS, superior sagittal sinus

Asymmetrical hydrocephalus

Asymmetrical hydrocephalus occurs due to unilateral obstruction of the foramen of Monro (Figures 5.12 and 5.13), an interhemispheric cyst (Figure 5.14), agenesis or dysgenesis of the corpus callosum (Figures 5.15 and 5.16), cerebral hemorrhage and/or encephalopathy in a single hemisphere. Outcome may be normal, but fetuses with increasing unilateral ventriculomegaly and cases associated with other brain abnormalities tend to have a poor neurological outcome[3].

X-linked hydrocephalus

X-linked hydrocephalus (HSAS, hydrocephalus due to stenosis of the aqueduct of Sylvius), mental retardation, aphasia, shuffling gait, adducted thumbs (MASA) syndrome, X-linked complicated spastic paraparesis (SP1) and X-linked corpus callosum agenesis (ACC) are all due to mutations in the L1 gene[4]. The gene encoding L1 is located near the telomere of the long arm of the X chromosome in Xq28. Therefore, it was suggested that this clinical syndrome be referred to by the acronym CRASH, for corpus callosum hypoplasia, retardation, adducted thumbs, spastic paraplegia and hydrocephalus[4]. It has been reported that mutations which produce truncations in the extracellular domain of the L1 protein are more likely to produce severe hydrocephalus, grave mental retardation or early death than point mutations in the extracellular domain or mutations affecting only the cytoplasmic domain of the protein[5]. For the families, prenatal CNS diagnosis in male infants is important. Prenatal images of CRASH syndrome are shown in Figures 5.17–5.20. A morphology-based approach becomes feasible between postmenstrual weeks 15 and 20. Prior to this gestational age, the diagnosis should rely on molecular biology tests[6].

Borderline (mild) ventriculomegaly

Borderline ventriculomegaly (Figures 5.21 and 5.22) is defined as a width of the atrium of the lateral cerebral ventricles of 10–15 mm. The majority of cases with prenatally detected isolated mild ventriculomegaly are developmentally normal[7]. Pilu and his colleagues[8] reviewed 234 cases of borderline ventriculomegaly including an abnormal outcome in 22.8% and concluded that borderline ventriculomegaly carries an increased risk of cerebral maldevelopment, delayed neurological development and, possibly, chromosomal aberrations.

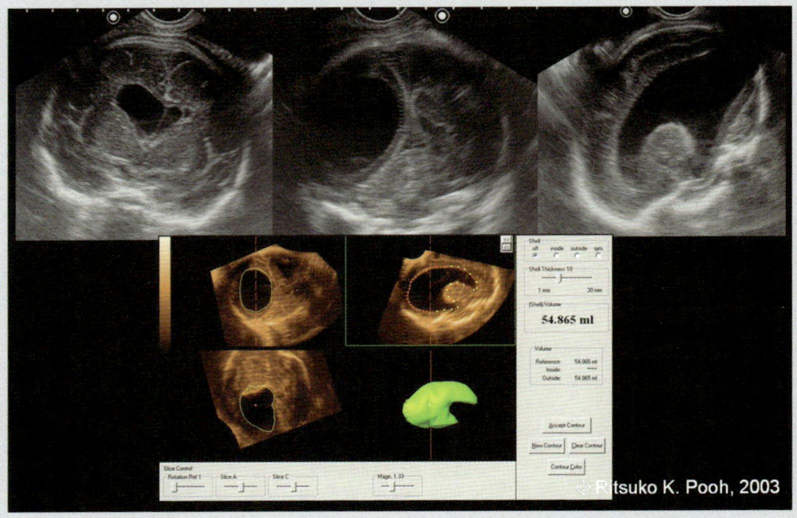

Figure 5.12 Fetal ultrasound images of unilateral ventriculomegaly at 30 weeks of gestation. Upper and middle, anterior and posterior coronal images; upper right, parasagittal image; lower, three-dimensional volume extraction images and volume calculation of the enlarged ventricle. Postnatal treatment in this case is shown in Figure 5.34

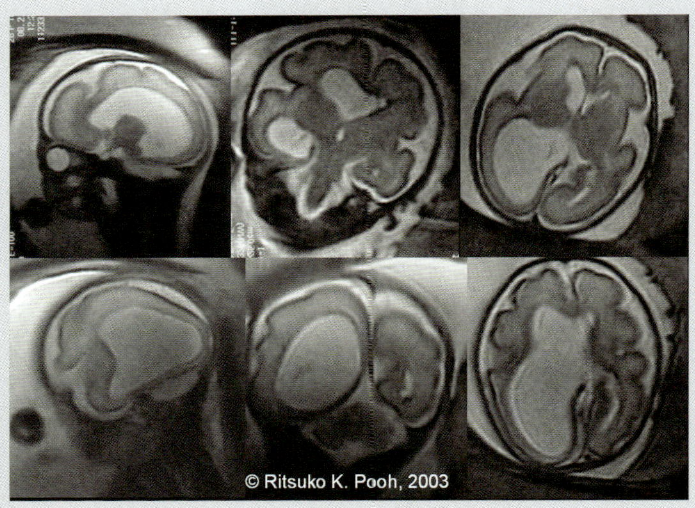

Figure 5.13 Fetal magnetic resonance images of unilateral ventriculomegaly at 29 weeks of gestation (same case as shown in Figure 5.12). Left, sagittal images; middle, coronal images; right, axial images. In this case, hemispheric asymmetry is very mild. The cause of unilateral ventriculomegaly may be unilateral obstruction or stenosis of the foramen of Monro. Ventriculomegaly gradually progressed into unilateral hydrocephalus *in utero*. Postnatal treatment in this case is shown in Figure 5.34. Postnatal prognosis has been good for 17 months

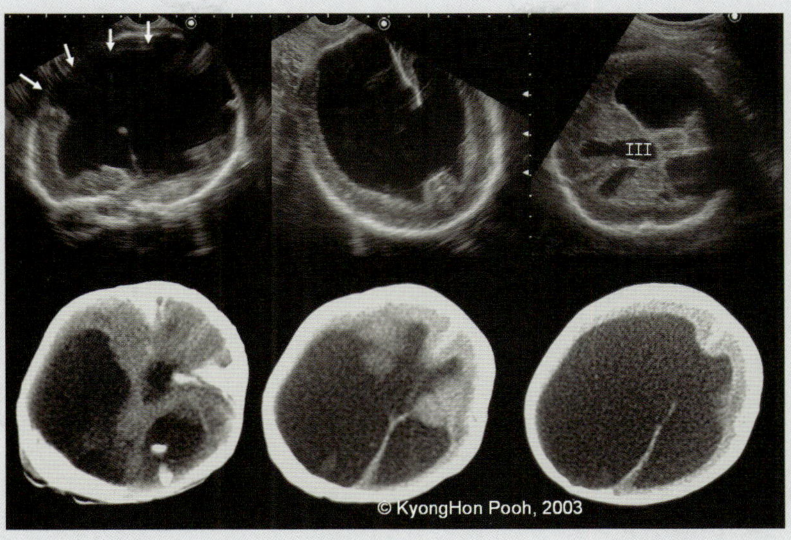

Figure 5.14 Fetal ultrasound image of asymmetrical hydrocephalus and postnatal computer tomography images at 31 weeks of gestation. Upper, ultrasound sagittal and axial images. Agenesis of the corpus callosum, interhemispheric cyst (arrows) fused with lateral ventricles and asymmetrical hydrocephaly with third ventriculomegaly (III) are complications. This case was complicated by congenital muscular dystrophy and postnatal prognosis was poor

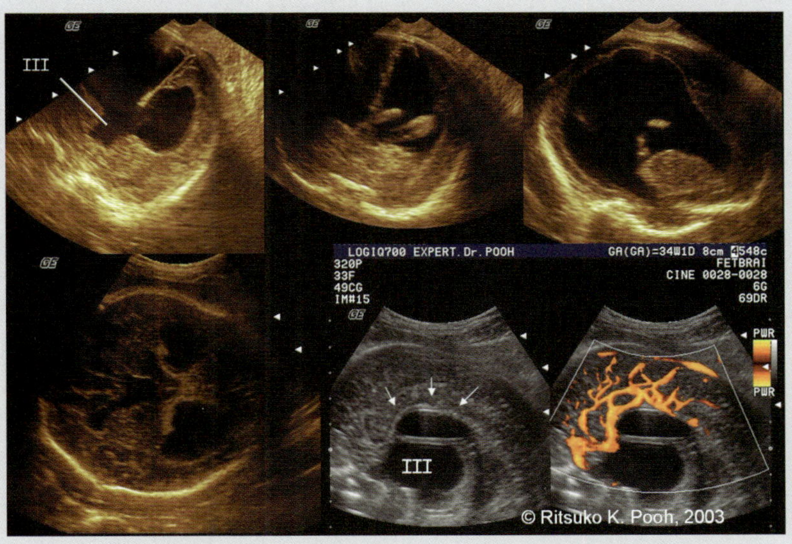

Figure 5.15 Fetal ultrasound images of hydrocephalus with hypogenesis of the corpus callosum at 34 weeks of gestation. Upper left and middle, coronal images; upper right, parasagittal images; lower left, axial image; lower middle and right, sagittal B-mode and power Doppler images. The corpus callosum is very thin but observable (arrows) with intact pericallosal arteries. Postnatal treatment in this case is shown in Figures 5.31–33

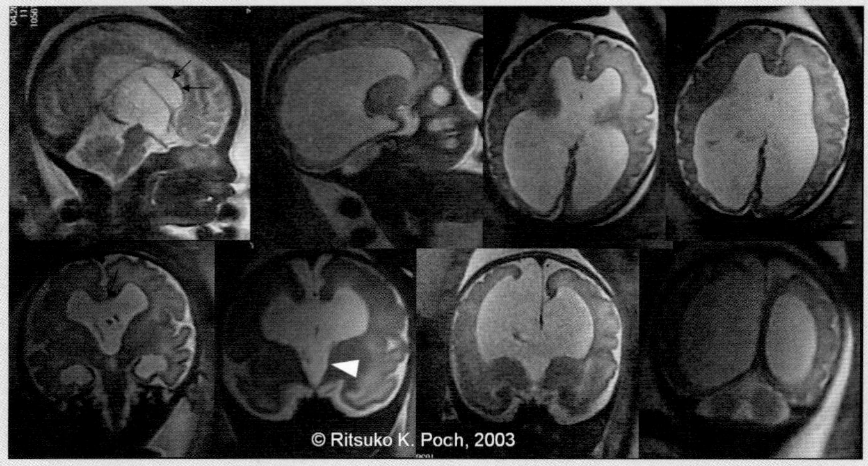

Figure 5.16 Fetal magnetic resonance images (MRI) of hydrocephalus with hypogenesis of the corpus callosum at 33 weeks of gestation (same case as shown in Figure 5.15). Upper, sagittal and axial MRIs; lower, serial axial images. Hypogenesis of the corpus callosum (arrows) is demonstrated. The bilateral ventricles and third ventricle (arrowhead) are fused because of destroyed septum pellucidum and dilated foramen of Monro. Mild asymmetry between the lateral ventricles may be due to posterior half agenesis of the corpus callosum. Postnatal treatment in this case is shown in Figures 5.31–33. The postnatal course has been good for 2 years

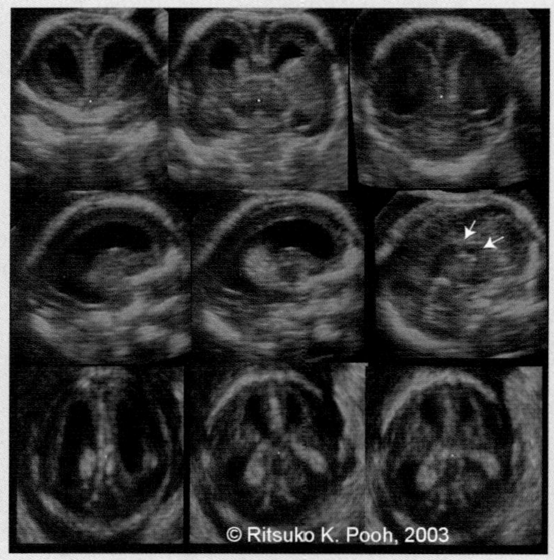

Figure 5.17 Ventriculomegaly at 20 weeks of gestation (X-linked hydrocephalus). Serial coronal (upper), sagittal (middle) and axial (lower) ultrasound images. This male fetus is a sibling of an 8-year-old boy with congenital hydrocephalus, adducted thumbs, aphasia and severe disability. The transvaginal sonograms show moderate ventriculomegaly with intact subarachnoid space. Partial agenesis of the corpus callosum is also present (arrows)

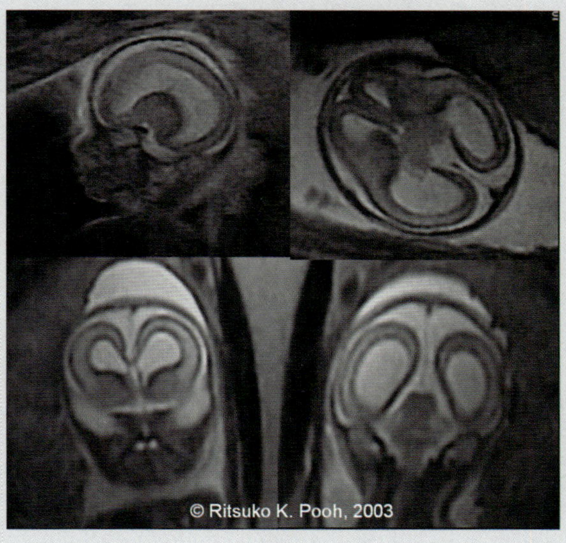

Figure 5.18 Magnetic resonance images of ventriculomegaly at 20 weeks of gestation (X-linked hydrocephalus; same case as shown in Figure 5.17). Upper left, parasagittal; upper right, axial; lower, coronal ultrasound images. Moderate ventriculomegaly and intact subarachnoid space are demonstrated. The subarachnoid space appears normal; therefore, this is ventriculomegaly not yet hydrocephalus

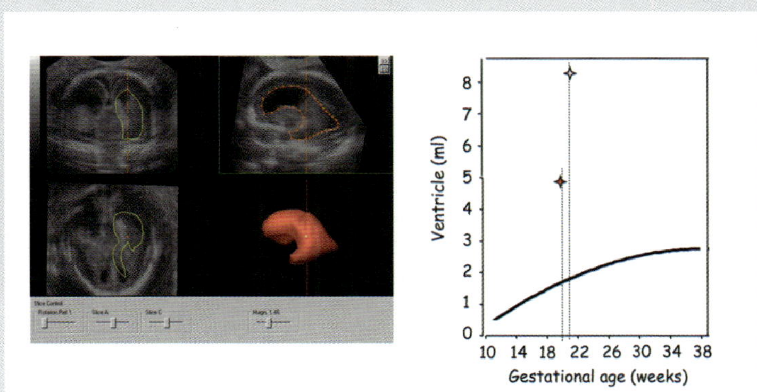

Figure 5.19 Lateral ventricular volume analysis in X-linked hydrocephalus (same case as shown in Figures 5.17 and 5.18). Volume calculation of the lateral ventricle was carried out. The result (right) shows rapid progression of lateral ventricular enlargement

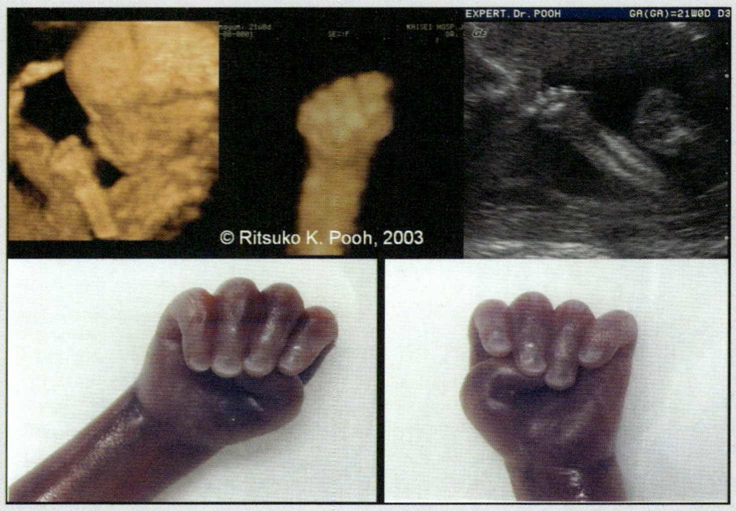

Figure 5.20 Adducted thumbs associated with ventriculomegaly at 21 weeks of gestation (X-linked hydrocephalus, same case as shown in Figures 5.17–5.19). Three-dimensional ultrasound images (upper left and middle) indicate adducted thumbs. Two-dimensional image (upper right) shows the thumb inside the four digits. Pregnancy was terminated at 21 weeks. Lower, external appearance of the hands of the same aborted fetus. Lower photographs courtesy of Dr M. Tanemura

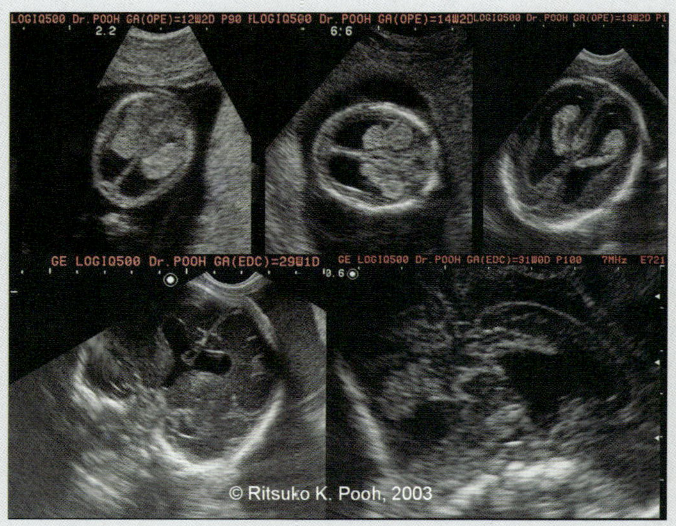

Figure 5.21 Mild ventriculomegaly detected from early pregnancy. Upper left, axial image at 12 weeks; posterior deviation of the choroid plexus is seen. Upper middle, 14 weeks; more conspicuous deviation of the choroid plexus. Upper right, 19 weeks; mild ventriculomegaly with deviated choroid plexus is observed. Lower left, anterior coronal image at 29 weeks; enlargement of the anterior horns with third ventriculomegaly is demonstrated. Lower right, sagittal image at 31 weeks; enlargement of the third ventricle; Dandy–Walker variant is also present in this case. The postnatal prognosis has been quite good for 3 years

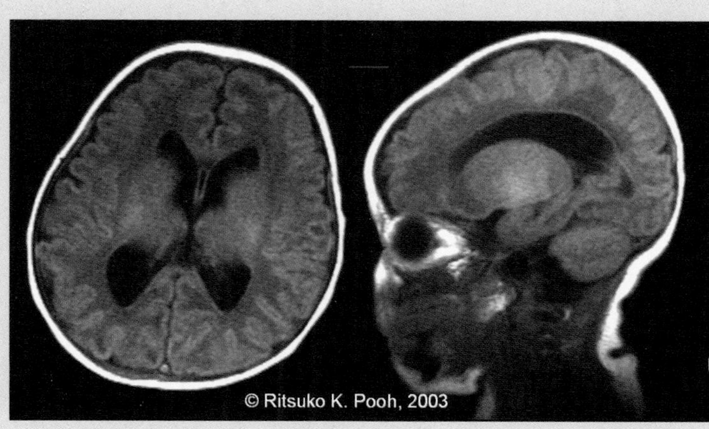

Figure 5.22 Postnatal magnetic resonance images of mild ventriculomegaly (same case as shown in Figure 5.21). Mild ventriculomegaly was indicated from early pregnancy. However, no progression was seen and the prognosis was good

NEUROSURGICAL MANAGEMENT OF HYDROCEPHALUS

Classification of congenital hydrocephalus

The term 'hydrocephalus' does not identify a specified disease, but is a generic term which means a serial pathological condition due to abnormal circulation of CSF. The method of treatment for hydrocephalus should be selected according to age of onset and symptoms. Congenital hydrocephalus is classified by causes into three categories which disturb the CSF circulation pathway (see Figure 2.13, normal CSF circulation), simple hydrocephalus, dysgenetic hydrocephalus and secondary hydrocephalus.

(1) *Simple hydrocephalus* Simple hydrocephalus, caused by a developmental abnormality which is localized within the CSF circulation pathway, includes aqueductal stenosis, atresia of Monro's foramen and maldevelopment of arachnoid granulation. Types of hydrocephalus due to various obstructive sites of CSF flow are shown in Figure 5.23. Hydrocephalus due to maldevelopment of arachnoid granulation is shown in Figure 5.24.

(2) *Dysgenetic hydrocephalus* Dysgenetic hydrocephalus indicates hydrocephalus as a result of a cerebral developmental disorder at an early developmental stage and includes hydranencephaly, holoprosencephaly, porencephaly, schizencephaly, Dandy–Walker malformation, dysraphism and Chiari malformation (see Chapters 6 and 7).

(3) *Secondary hydrocephalus* Secondary hydrocephalus is a generic term indicating hydrocephalus caused by an intracranial pathological condition, such as a brain tumor (Figure 5.25), intracranial infection and intracranial hemorrhage.

Neurosurgical treatment of hydrocephalus

Miniature Ommaya reservoir

The main treatment of congenital hydrocephalus is the shunt procedure. It is preferable to place the shunting tube immediately after birth. However, risk of shunt complications exists in cases of posthemorrhagic hydrocephalus[9] with high concentrations of CSF protein, in cases of myelomeningocele with a high risk of cerebrospinal infection, or in premature neonates with thin and brittle skin. A miniature Ommaya reservoir[10,11] (Figure 5.26) can be placed as the first treatment until the shunt procedure and

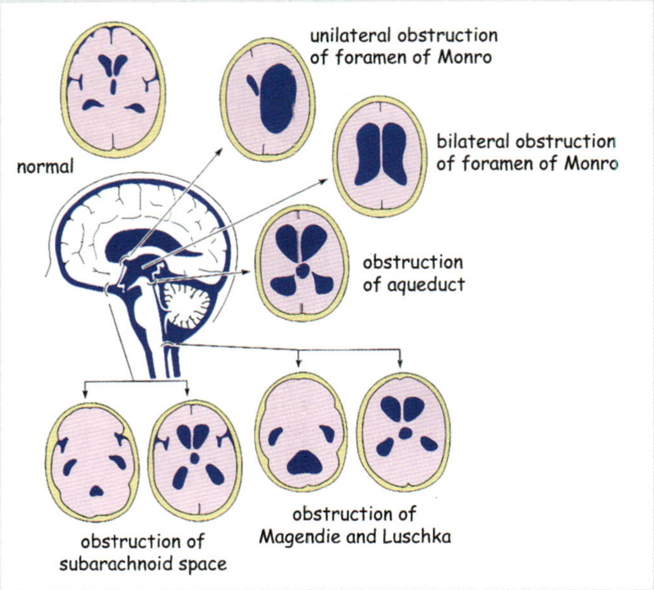

Figure 5.23 Types of hydrocephalus due to various obstructive sites of cerebrospinal fluid flow. From *Handbook on Hydrocephalus for Patients*, Research Committee of Intractable Hydrocephalus, Japanese Ministry of Health and Welfare, ©1993, with permission. Schema courtesy of chairman of the Committee, Professor K. Mori

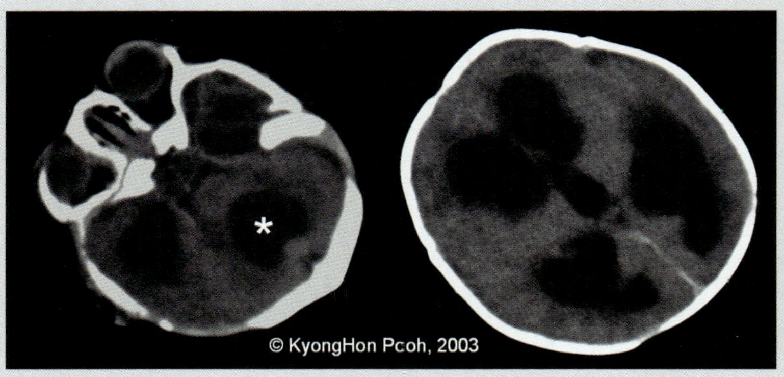

Figure 5.24 Hydrocephalus due to maldevelopment of arachnoid granulation. Disturbance of absorption of cerebrospinal fluid due to maldevelopment of arachnoid granulation, results in an enlargement of all ventricles. Note the IVth ventriculomegaly (asterisk), which cannot be seen in cases with other types of hydrocephalus

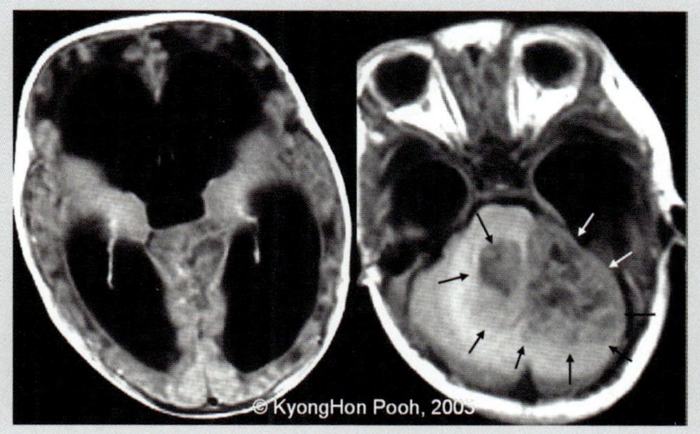

Figure 5.25 Secondary obstructive hydrocephalus. Left, magnetic resonance axial image. Symmetrical hydrocephalus is demonstrated. Hydrocephalus is secondarily caused by a brain tumor filling the fourth ventricle (right, arrows)

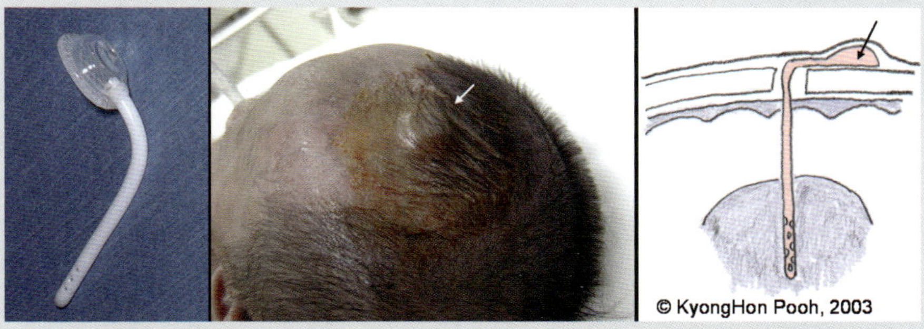

Figure 5.26 Miniature Ommaya reservoir. Left, photograph of miniature Ommaya reservoir. Middle, subcutaneous placement of a reservoir (white arrow) in a case of hydrocephalus. Reliable fluid reduction can be carried out by percutaneous puncture. Right, schema of Ommaya reservoir; intermittent drainage is possible from the reservoir (black arrow)

it is possible to control the intracranial pressure (ICP) by percutaneous puncture and intermittent drainage of CSF through a reservoir. In some cases of posthemorrhagic hydrocephalus, intermittent drainage leads to normalization of the CSF flow pathway and there is no need for the shunt procedure (Figure 5.27).

Shunt procedure

The shunt operation includes the ventriculoperitoneal shunt (VP shunt), the ventriculoatrial shunt (VA shunt) and the lumboperitoneal shunt (Figure 5.28). The ventriculoperitoneal shunt is the most popular procedure. Effectiveness of the shunt

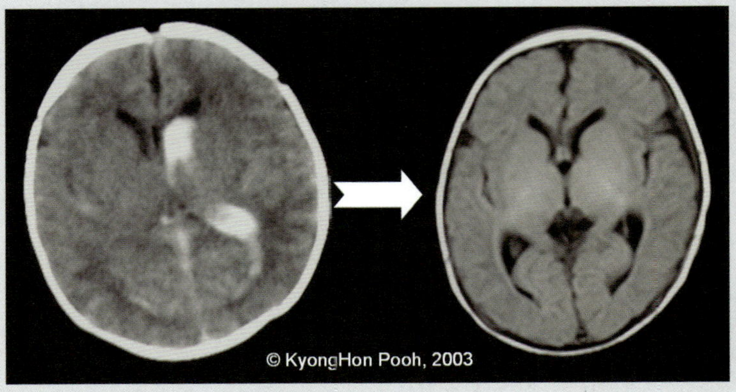

Figure 5.27 Treatment of ventriculomegaly due to intraventricular hemorrhage. Left, unilateral intraventricular hemorrhage in a neonate. Due to the gradual progression of hydrocephalus, an Ommaya reservoir was placed. Intermittent drainage of the cerebrospinal fluid resulted in remission of the hydrocephalus. Right, magnetic resonance image after treatment

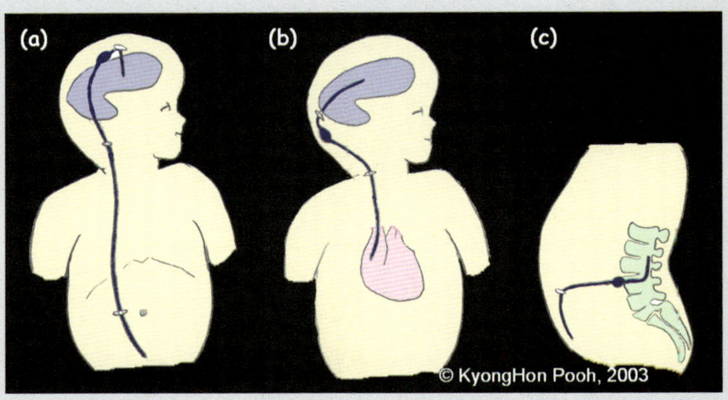

Figure 5.28 Shunt procedure. (a)Ventriculoperitoneal shunt. (b) Ventriculoatrial shunt. (c) Lumboperitoneal shunt. The ventriculoperitoneal shunt (a) is the most popular shunt procedure

procedure for congenital hydrocephalus (Figures 5.29–5.34) has been proven. However, it is known that there are various complications of shunting, such as shunt infection, obstruction of the shunt tube, over-drainage, under-drainage and slit ventricle syndrome (Figure 5.35). To reduce these complications, various types of shunt devices, such as an anti-siphon device or pressure programmable valve shunt device have been developed.

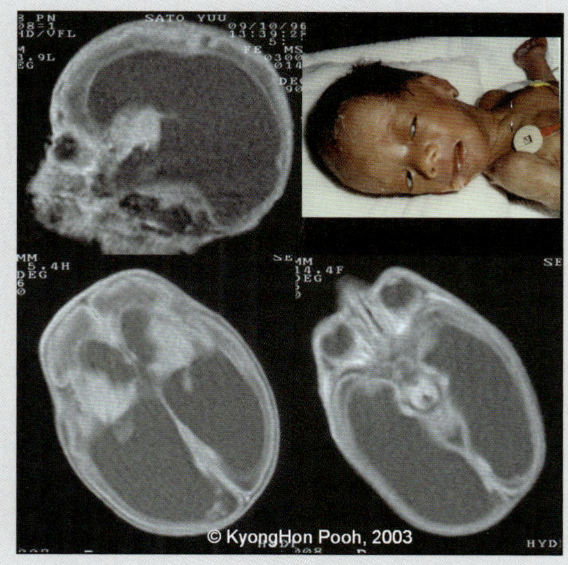

Figure 5.29 Congenital hydrocephalus (referral at 39th postnatal day, before treatment). Upper left, magnetic resonance (MR) sagittal image of severe hydrocephalus. Lower, MR axial images of symmetrical hydrocephalus. Upper right, the infant face and head

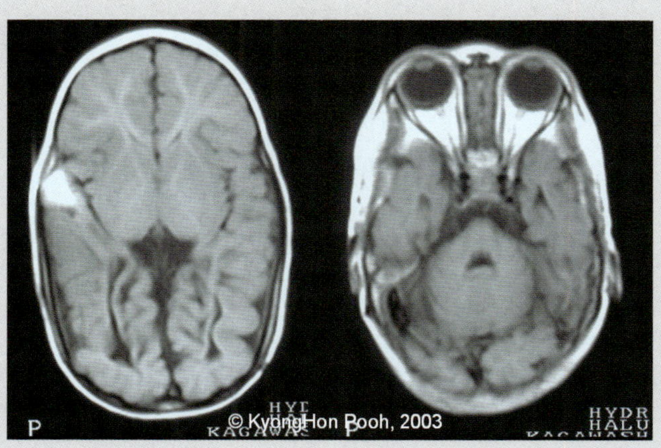

Figure 5.30 Postoperative magnetic resonance images (same case as shown in Figure 5.29, 2 years after the operation). After a ventriculoperitoneal shunt, the hydrocephalus was well controlled

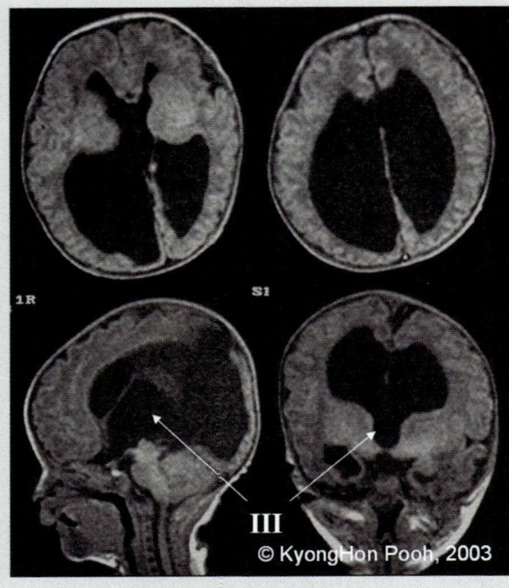

Figure 5.31 Hydrocephalus due to aqueductal stenosis (neonatal magnetic resonance image (MRI), before treatment). Prenatal ultrasound and MRIs are shown in Figures 5.15 and 5.16. Upper, axial sections; bilateral hydrocephalus with mild asymmetry. Lower left, sagittal section; hypogenesis of the corpus callosum is a complication in this case. Lower right, coronal section; remarkable enlargement of the bilateral lateral ventricles and third ventricle (III) is demonstrated. The aqueduct is not depicted in the sagittal section

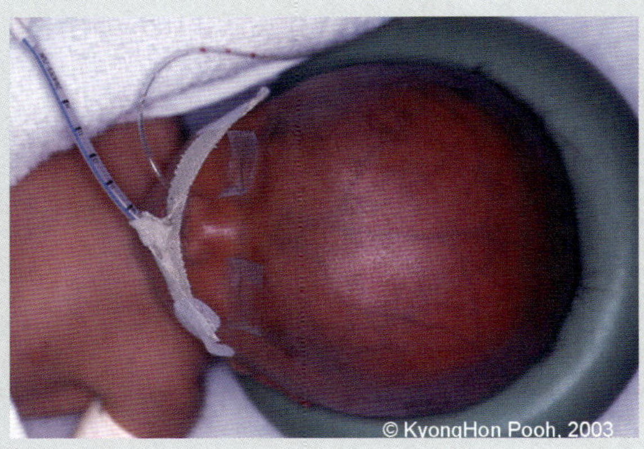

Figure 5.32 Photograph of the head and face of an infant with hydrocephalus (same case as shown in Figure 5.31). Note the remarkable increase of the head circumference, engorgement of the scalp venous vessels and the bulge of the anterior fontanelle

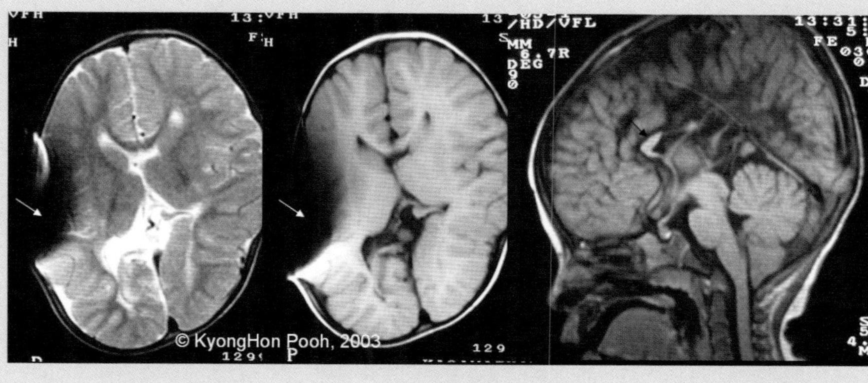

Figure 5.33 Postoperative magnetic resonance images (same infant as shown in Figures 5.31 and 5.32) after a ventriculoperitoneal shunt. Left and middle, axial section. Artifact (white arrow) is seen due to the pressure programmable shunt valve. Right, sagittal section. Hypogenesis of the corpus callosum is demonstrated (black arrow). Postoperative prognosis has been good for 2 years

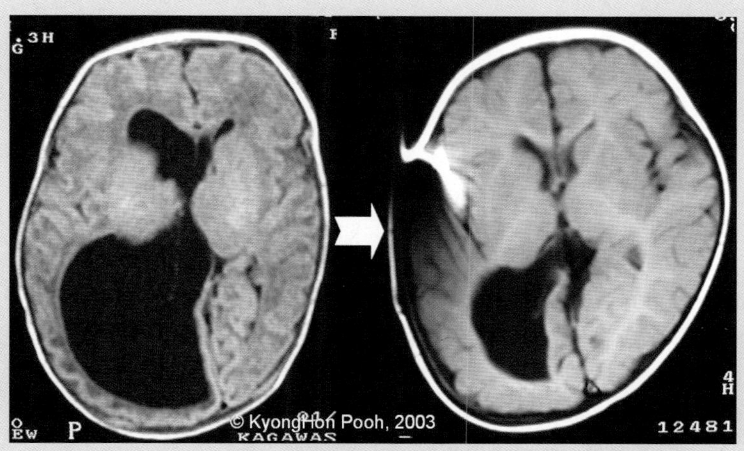

Figure 5.34 Treatment of unilateral hydrocephalus. Prenatal ultrasound and magnetic resonance images (MRIs) are shown in Figures 5.12 and 5.13. Left, neonatal MRI before treatment. Unilateral hydrocephalus is demonstrated due to obstruction of the foramen of Monro unilaterally. Right, after a ventriculoperitoneal shunt. Unilateral ventriculomegaly still exists; however, postnatal development has been normal and no neurological deficiencies have been seen for 17 months

Neuroendoscopy

Third ventriculostomy by neuroendoscopy (Figures 5.36–5.38) has recently been performed in children with obstructive hydrocephalus, and the number of shunt-independent cases has increased. It has been controversial, however, as to whether infants under than the age of 1 year have a higher risk of treatment failure after neuroendoscopic procedures than older children. Some conclude that neuroendoscopy presents an effective alternative for the treatment of hydrocephalus in cases under the age of 1 year[12].

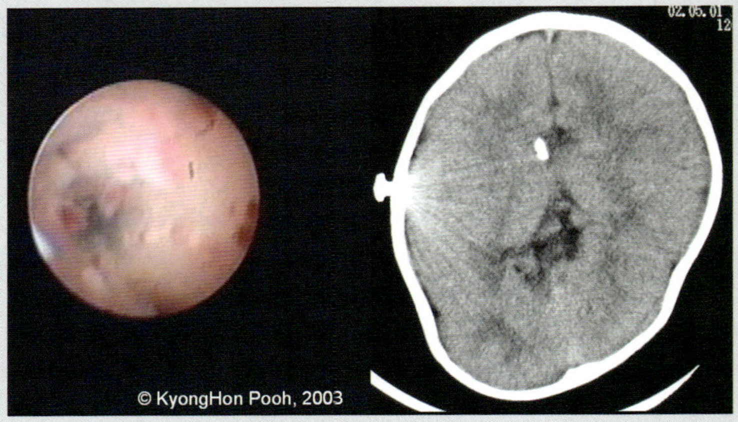

Figure 5.35 Slit ventricle. Left, neuroendoscopic view of a slit lateral ventricle. Right, CT axial image. Continuation of overdrainage by the shunt procedure leads to these slit-like ventricles, which cause shunt tube obstruction. To avoid slit ventricles, an antisiphon device and/or a pressure programmable valve have been developed

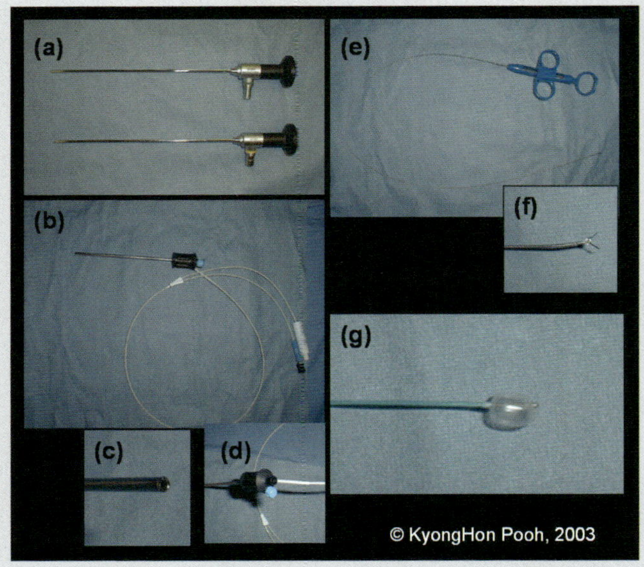

Figure 5.36 Neuroendoscope and its instruments. (a) Rigid endoscopes for observation. (b) Rigid endoscope for operation. (c) Viewer side of endoscope (b). (d) Operational side of endoscope (b). (e) Forceps. (f) The head of forceps. (g) Balloon catheter

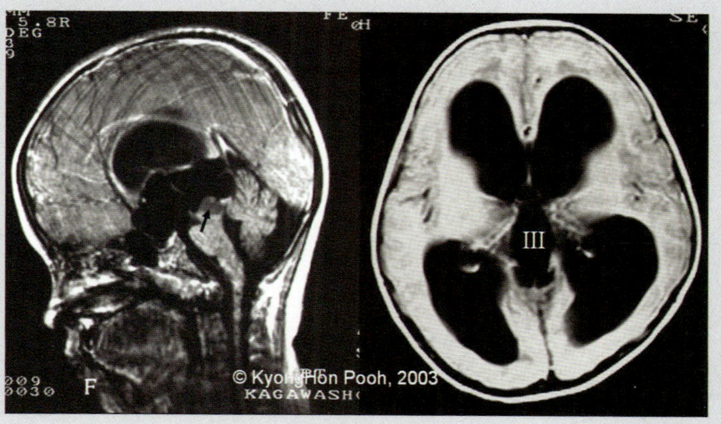

Figure 5.37 Obstructive hydrocephalus by tumor of the aqueduct. Left, magnetic resonance (MR) sagittal image. An aqueductal tumor (black arrow) causes enlargement of the third ventricle and bilateral lateral ventricles. Right, MR axial image. Symmetrical hydrocephalus and third ventriculomegaly (III) are demonstrated. This condition is an indication for third ventriculostomy by neuroendoscopy

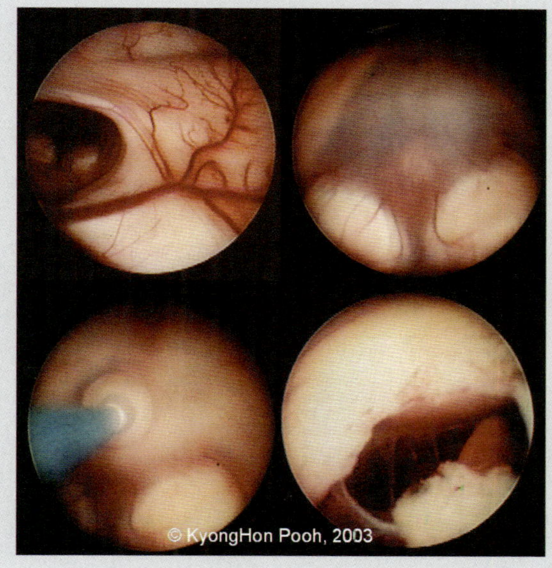

Figure 5.38 Neuroendoscopic views in third ventriculostomy. Upper left, view of the foramen of Monro through the lateral ventricle. Upper right, floor of the third ventricle. Lower left, dilatation of the stoma by ballooning. Lower right, view of the basilar artery through the dilated stoma

However, third ventriculostomy does not seem to be effective in neonates and small infants because of the prematurity of their CSF absorption ability.

REFERENCES

1. Pooh RK, Maeda K, Pooh KH, *et al.* Sonographic assessment of the fetal brain morphology. *Prenat Neonat Med* 1999;4:18–38
2. Pooh RK, Pooh KH, Nakagawa Y, *et al.* Transvaginal Doppler assessment of fetal intracranial venous flow. *Obstet Gynecol* 1999;93:697–701
3. Durfee SM, Kim FM, Benson CB. Postnatal outcome of fetuses with the prenatal diagnosis of asymmetric hydrocephalus. *J Ultrasound Med* 2001;20:263–8
4. Fransen E, Lemmon V, Van Camp G, *et al.* CRASH syndrome: clinical spectrum of corpus callosum hypoplasia, retardation, adducted thumbs, spastic paraparesis and hydrocephalus due to mutations in one single gene, L1. *Eur J Hum Genet* 1995;3:273–84
5. Yamasaki M, Thompson P, Lemmon V. CRASH syndrome: mutations in L1CAM correlate with severity of the disease. *Neuropediatrics* 1997;28:175–8
6. Timor-Tritsch IE, Monteagudo A, Haratz-Rubinstein N, *et al.* Transvaginal sonographic detection of adducted thumbs, hydrocephalus, and agenesis of the corpus callosum at 22 postmenstrual weeks: the masa spectrum or L1 spectrum. A case report and review of the literature. *Prenat Diagn* 1996;16:543–8
7. Patel MD, Filly AL, Hersh DR, *et al.* Isolated mild fetal cerebral ventriculomegaly: clinical course and outcome. *Radiology* 1994;192:759–64
8. Pilu G, Falco P, Gabrielli S, *et al.* The clinical significance of fetal isolated cerebral borderline ventriculomegaly: report of 31 cases and review of the literature. *Ultrasound Obstet Gynecol* 1999;14:320–6
9. Taylor AG, Peter JC. Advantages of delayed VP shunting in post-haemorrhagic hydrocephalus seen in low-birth-weight infants. *Childs Nerv Syst* 2001;17:328–33
10. Wakayama A, Morimoto K, Kitajima H, *et al.* Extremely low birth-weight infant with hydrocephalus; management of hydrocephalus using a miniature Ommaya's reservoir. *No Shinkei Geka* 1991;19:795–800
11. Morimoto K, Hayakawa T, Yoshimine T, *et al.* Two-step procedure for early neonatal surgery of fetal hydrocephalus. *Neurol Med Chir* 1993;33:158–65
12. Fritsch MJ, Mehdorn M. Endoscopic intraventricular surgery for treatment of hydrocephalus and loculated CSF space in children less than one year of age. *Pediatr Neurosurg* 2002;36:183–8

6

Congenital brain anomalies

R.K. Pooh and K.H. Pooh

DYSRAPHISM

This includes disorders of neurulation and neural tube formation.

Spina bifida (Figures 6.1–6.23)

Prevalence 0.22/1000 births[1]; overall neural tube defect (NTD), 0.58–1.17/1000 births[2–4]. Many authors have reported a remarkable reduction in prevalence of NTDs after using folic acid supplementation and fortification[1–5].

Definition

(1) Spina bifida aperta, manifest form of spina bifida, has been classified into four types: meningocele, myelomeningocele, myelocystocele and myeloschisis as shown in Figure 6.1. A three-dimensional CT of spina bifida is shown in Figures 6.19 and 6.20.

(2) Spina bifida occulta is a generic term for spinal bifida covered with normal skin tissue, and does not indicate spinal bifida which cannot be diagnosed by external appearance. Cutaneous

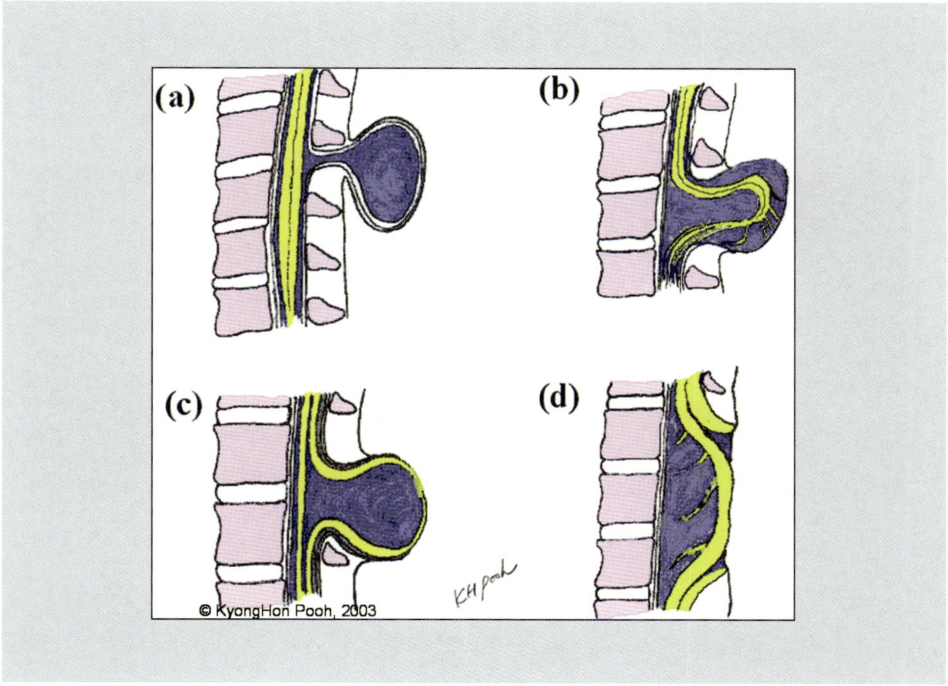

Figure 6.1 Classification of spina bifida aperta. (a) Meningocele, (b) myelomeningocele, (c) myelocystocele, (d) myeloschisis. The spinal cord is shown in yellow

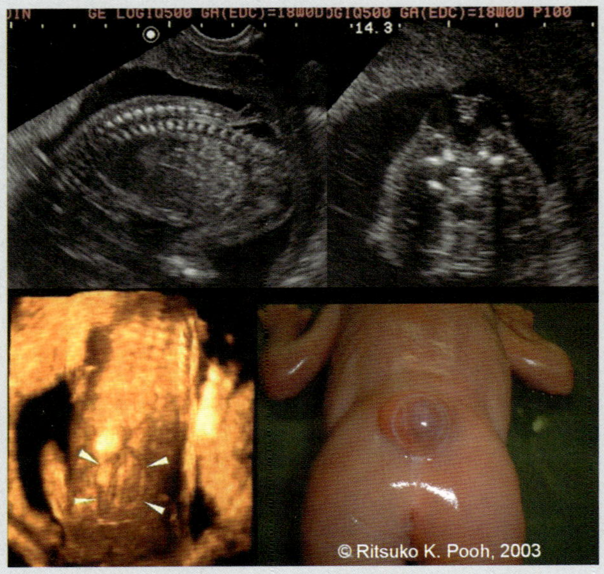

Figure 6.2 Myelomeningocele at 18 weeks of gestation. Upper left, sagittal ultrasound image. Note the spinal cord from spinal canal to the sac surface. Upper right, axial ultrasound image. Lower left, three-dimensional surface reconstruction of myelomeningocele. Lower right, external appearance of the aborted fetus at 19 weeks of gestation

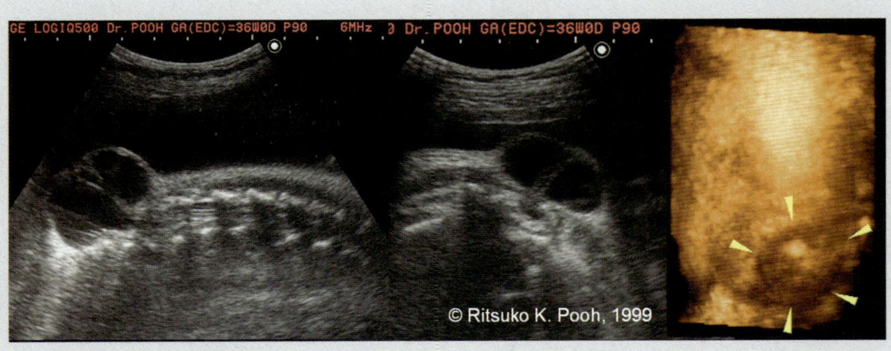

Figure 6.3 Myelomeningocele at 36 weeks of gestation. Sagittal image, axial image and three-dimensional surface reconstruction from the left side

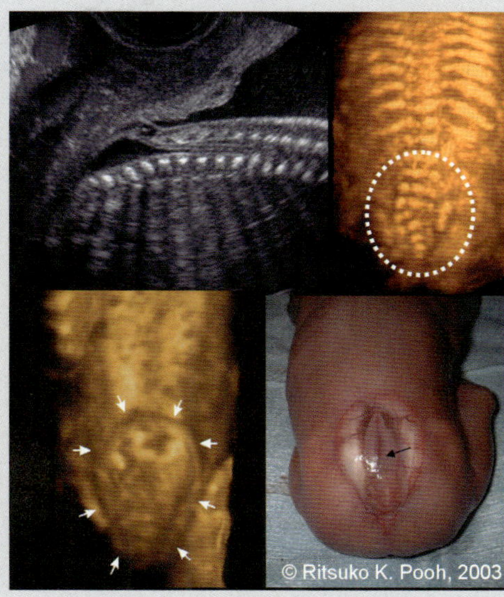

Figure 6.4 Prenatal ultrasound image of myelomeningocele and spina bifida at 20 weeks of gestation. Upper left, sagittal ultrasound image. The spinal cord protrudes into the sac surface from the spinal canal. Upper right, three-dimensional bony demonstration of lumbar spina bifida. Three-dimensional ultrasound shows the exact level of spina bifida. Lower left, three-dimensional surface reconstruction of a large myelomeningocele (white arrows). Lower right, external appearance of the aborted fetus at 21 weeks of gestation. Note the central canal of the spinal cord (black arrow) in a large myelomeningocele

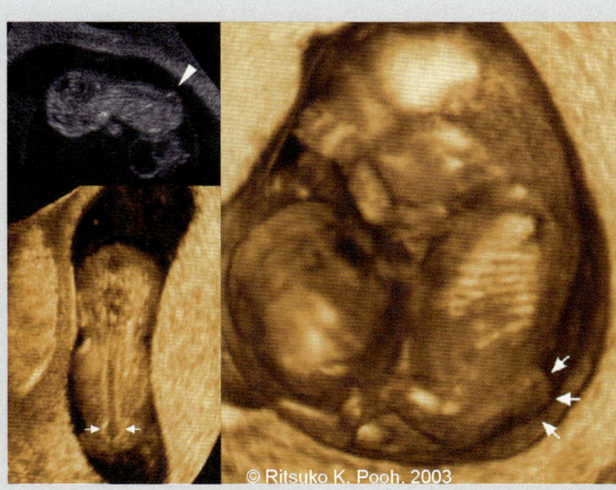

Figure 6.5 Prenatal ultrasound image of spina bifida at 9 and 12 weeks of gestation. Upper left, sagittal ultrasound image at 9 weeks and 3 days of gestation. Note the lumbar cystic lesion (arrowhead). Lower left, three-dimensional bony demonstration of lumbar spina bifida (arrows) at the same gestational age. Right, three-dimensional surface reconstruction of myelocystocele (arrows) at 12 weeks of gestation in the same fetus. This fetus has bladder extrophy. Termination of the pregnancy was carried out at 13 weeks and final diagnosis was omphalocele, bladder extrophy, imperforate anus and spine defect (OEIS)

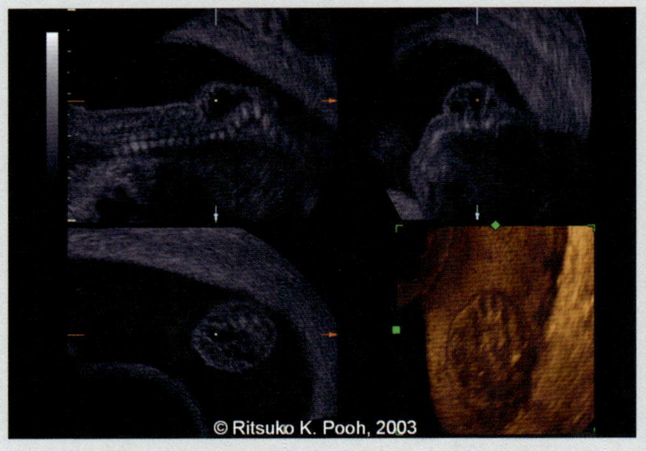

Figure 6.6 Three-dimensional ultrasound image of myelomeningocele with kyphosis at 16 weeks of gestation. Three orthogonal views and a surface reconstruction image. Upper left, sagittal ultrasound image. The spinal cord completely protrudes into the sac surface from the spinal canal and severe kyphosis is seen. Upper right, axial ultrasound view. Lower left, coronal ultrasound view of myelomeningocele. Lower right, surface reconstruction image of myelomeningocele

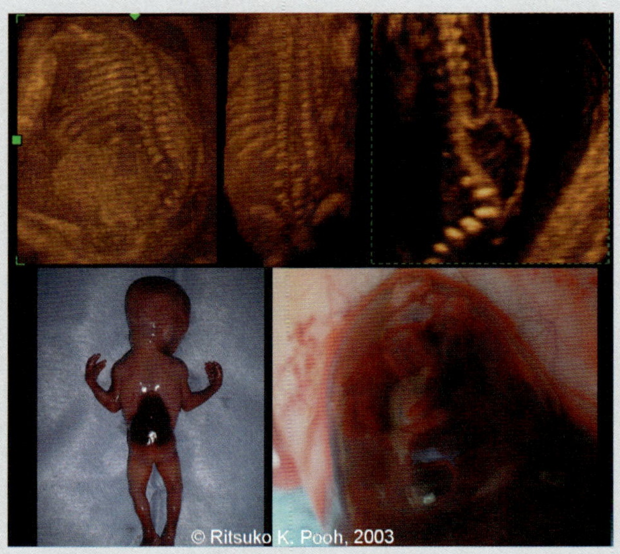

Figure 6.7 Bony structural images of kyphosis and spina bifida at 16 weeks of gestation (same case as shown in Figure 6.6). Upper left, middle, three-dimensional skeleton images of severe kyphosis and spina bifida. Upper right, inside view of kyphosis and myelomeningocele. Note the spinal cord and nerves inside the myelomeningocele. Lower left, external appearance of the aborted fetus at 17 weeks of gestation. Lower right, photograph of the myelomeningocele. Note the tortuous spinal cord inside the sac

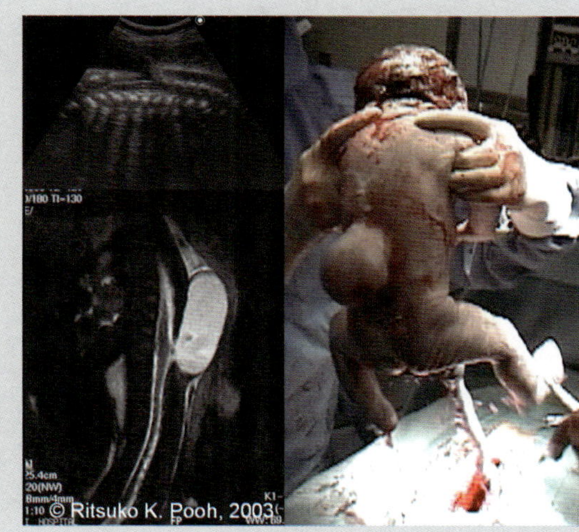

Figure 6.8 Meningocele in late pregnancy. Upper left, sagittal ultrasound image at 37 weeks of gestation. The spinal cord is located inside the spinal canal. Lower left, fetal magnetic resonance sagittal image. Right, external appearance of the neonate delivered by Cesarean section. The meningocele is completely covered by skin

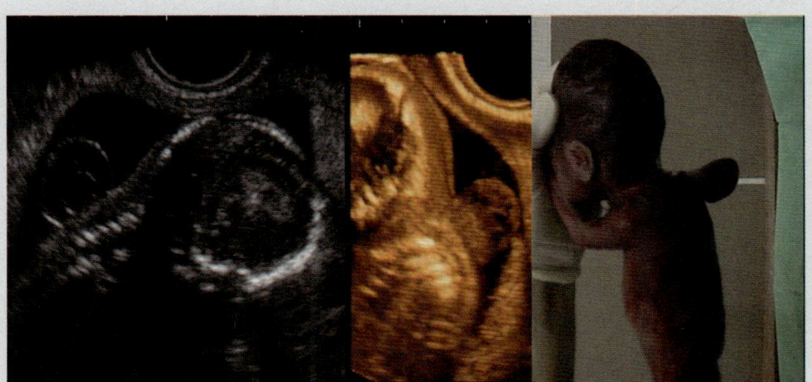

Figure 6.9 Cervical meningomyelocele at 16 weeks of gestation. Left, sagittal ultrasound image. A small cyst in the meningocele is demonstrated. The fetus has no nuchal translucency in the first trimester. Middle, three-dimensional surface reconstruction image. Right, external appearance of the aborted fetus at 23 weeks of gestation. Meningocele at the level of C6 with abnormal vertebrae between C3–4 and T1 was confirmed. Images and photograph courtesy of Dr G. Malinger

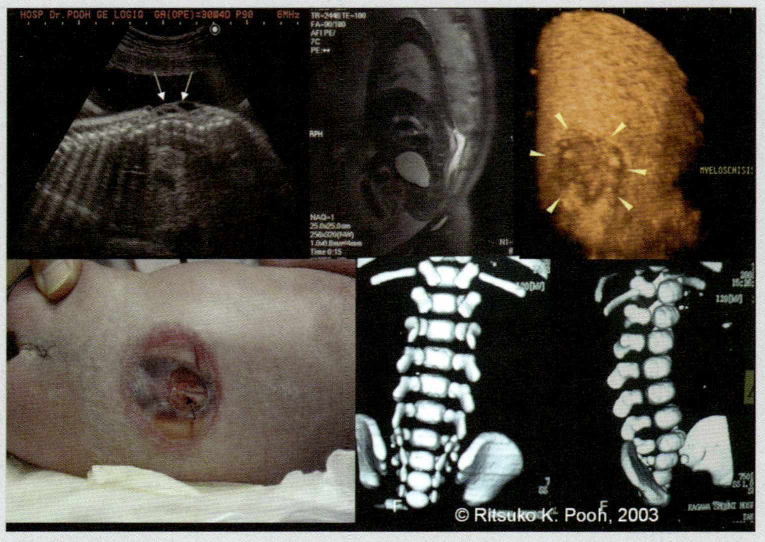

Figure 6.10 Myeloschisis with kyphosis. Upper left, sagittal ultrasound image of myeloschisis and kyphosis at 30 weeks of gestation; there is no cystic formation. The spinal cord (white arrows) is visible with a defect of the skin. Upper middle, fetal magnetic resonance sagittal image. Upper right, three-dimensional demonstration of the surface of myeloschisis. Lower left, external appearance of neonatal myeloschisis. The central canal of the spinal cord (black arrow) is visible. Lower middle and right, postnatal three-dimensional reconstruction CT images of spina bifida and kyphosis

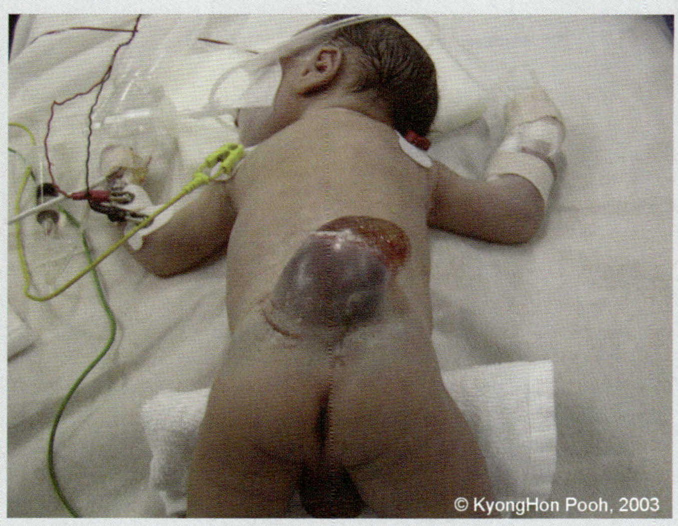

Figure 6.11 Myelomeningocele. The spinal cord and nerves are prolapsed into the sac. The sac, covered with a thin membrane, did not rupture

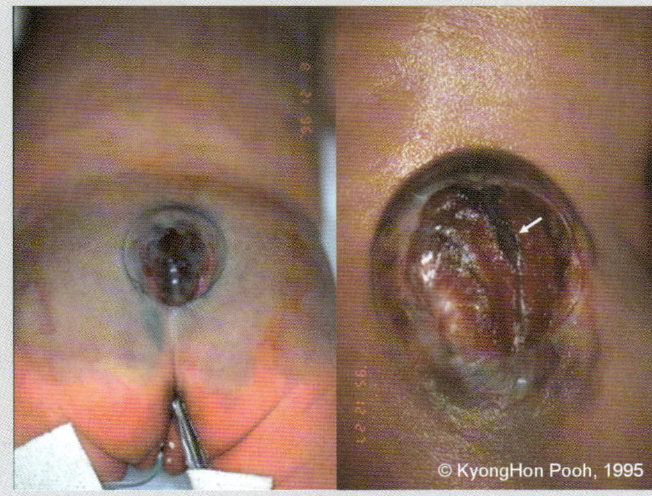

Figure 6.12 Myeloschisis. The black line on the center of the mass (arrow) indicates the central canal of the spinal cord

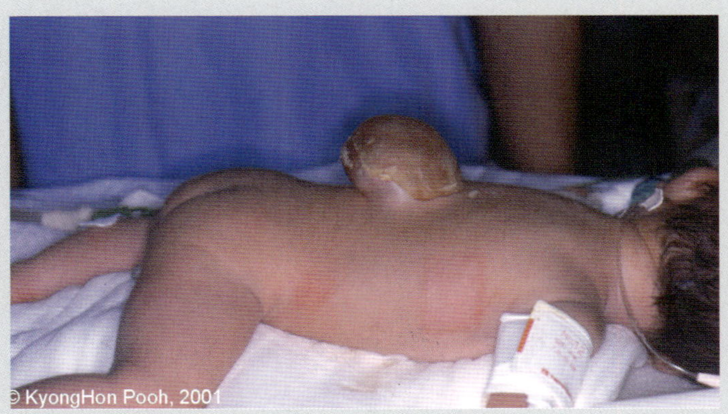

Figure 6.13 Thoracic meningocele. The wall of the cyst is thin but completely covered with skin

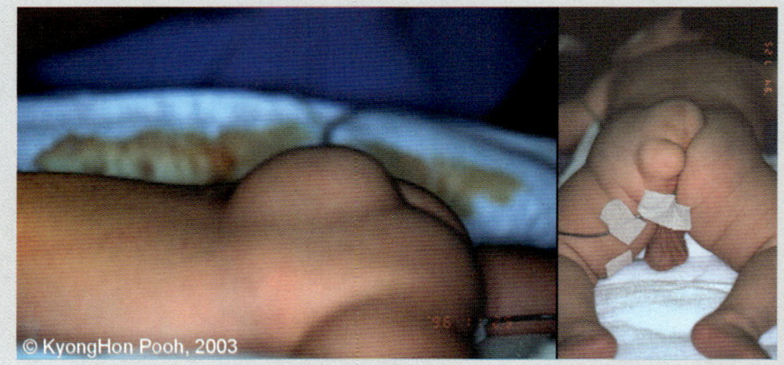

Figure 6.14 Spinal lipoma (spina bifida occulta) – lumbosacral subcutaneous lipoma. These spinal lipomas penetrate into the intradural space

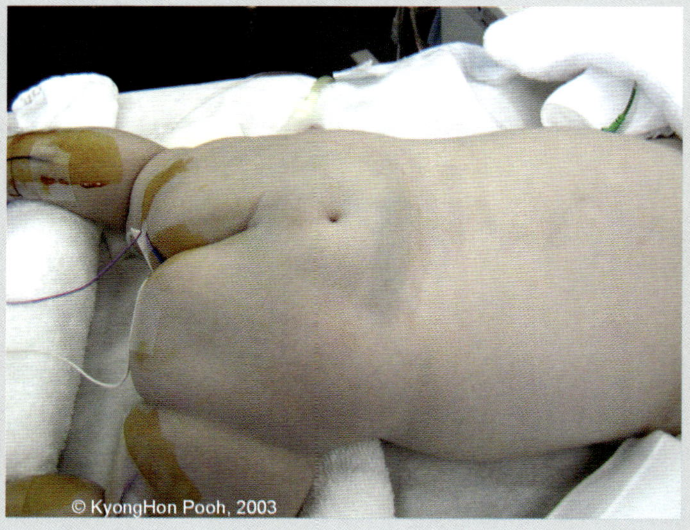

Figure 6.15 Spinal lipoma (spina bifida ccculta) with a dermal sinus. In this case, the dermal sinus is complicated by spinal lipoma

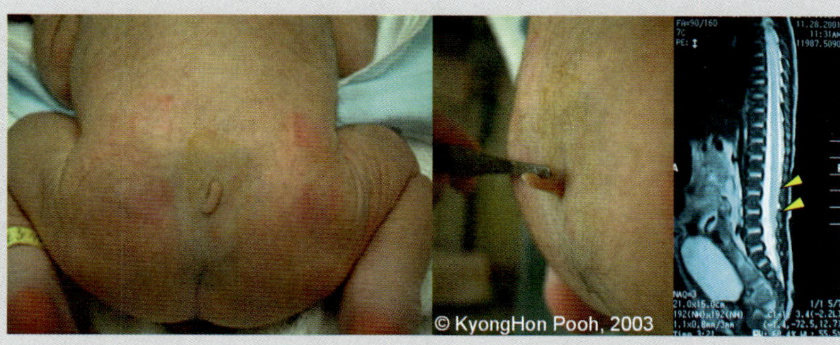

Figure 6.16 Skin appendage; spinal bifida occulta (neonate). Left, middle, external appearance of a human tail after birth. This small cutaneous abnormality is a sign of spina bifida occulta. Right, magnetic resonance sagittal image of a tethered cord in the same neonate. Note abnormal location of the spinal cord in the spinal canal (yellow arrows)

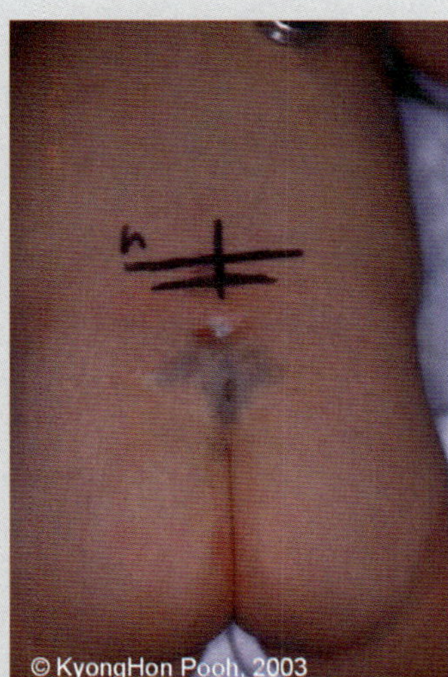

Figure 6.17 External appearance of a dermal sinus. Through the thin skin, the funicular stalk penetrates into the intradural space

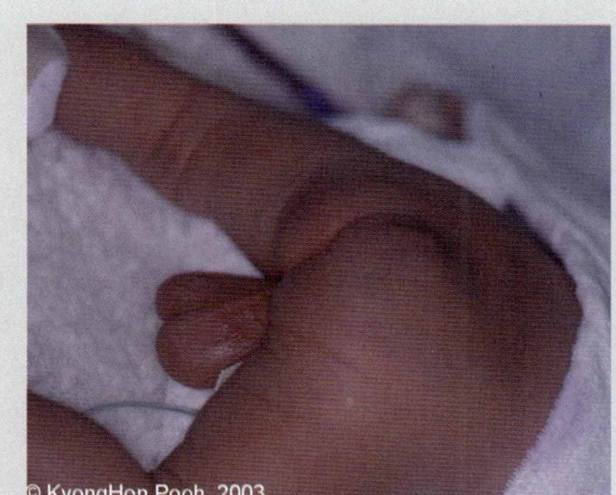

Figure 6.18 External appearance of sacrococcigeal teratoma. This disease should be differentiated from spinal lipoma

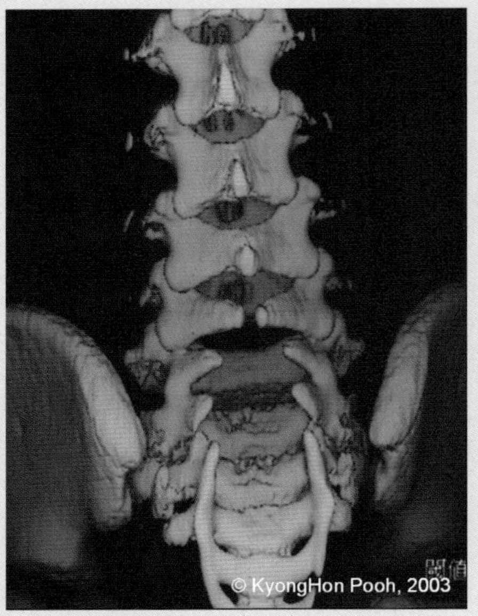

Figure 6.19 Three-dimensional reconstruction CT image of spina bifida. A defect of the lamina of the vertebrae is clearly demonstrated

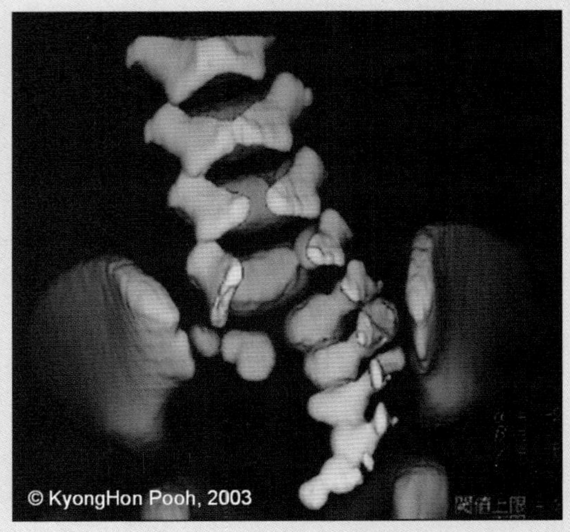

Figure 6.20 Three-dimensional reconstruction CT image of spina bifida. A partial defect of the sacral bone is demonstrated in a case of spinal lipoma

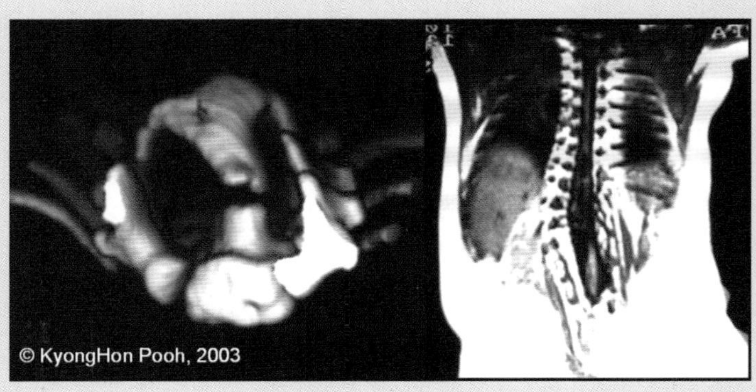

Figure 6.21 Diastematomyelia (split cord). Left, three-dimensional CT and (right) magnetic resonance image. The spinal cord is divided into two parts (split cord') by a chondro-osseous septum

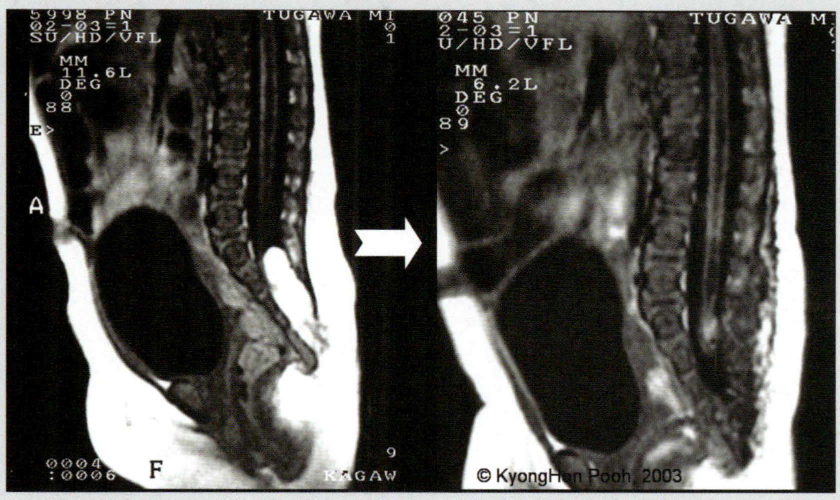

Figure 6.22 Magnetic resonance image of spinal lipoma (before and after operation). Left, before operation. A subcutaneous lipoma penetrates into the intradural space and adheres to the terminus of the spinal cord (cornus). In this case, dilatation of the central canal of the spinal cord is a complication. Right, magnetic resonance image after resection of the spinal lipoma

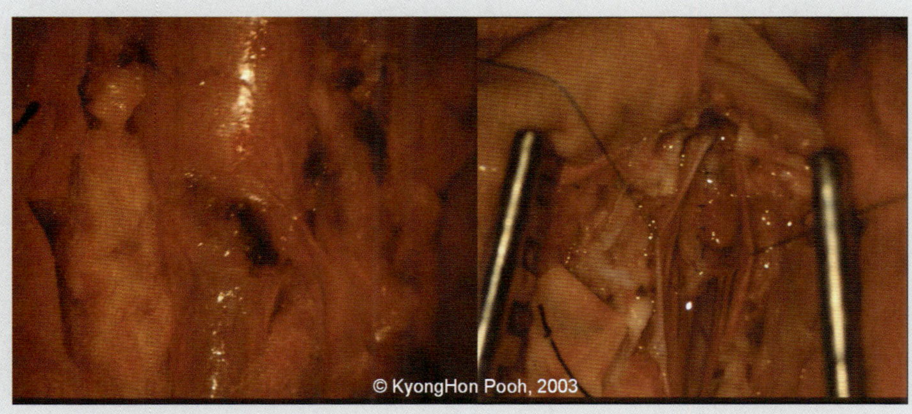

Figure 6.23 Spinal lipoma; intraoperative photograph. Left, a spinal lipoma, penetrating into the intradural space, is exposed. Right, repair of the cornus after resection of lipoma. The spinal nerves of the cauda equina can be seen

abnormalities near the spinal lesion are found: skin bulge (subcutaneous lipoma), dimple, hair tuft, pigmentation, skin appendage and hemangioma (Figures 6.13–6.17). In cases with thickened film terminale, dermal sinus or diastematomyelia (split cord malformation, Figure 6.21), abnormal tethering and fixation of the spinal cord occur.

Etiology Multifactorial inheritance, single mutant genes, autosomal recessive, chromosomal abnormalities (trisomy 18, 13), specific teratogens (valproic acid), maternal diabetes, environmental factors. Predominant in females.

Pathogenesis Spina bifida aperta is an impairment of neural tube closure; spina bifida occulta is due to a caudal neural tube malformation by the processes of canalization and retrogressive differentiation.

Associated anomalies Chiari type II malformation, hydrocephalus, scoliosis (above L2), polyhydramnios, additional non-CNS anomalies.

Prenatal diagnosis Figures 6.2–6.10; neonatal appearance, Figures 6.11–6.13.

Differential diagnosis Sacrococcygeal teratoma, Figure 6.18.

Prognosis Disturbance of motor, sensory and sphincter function. Depends on lesion levels. Below S1: able to walk unaided; above L2: wheelchair dependent; variable at intermediate level.

Recurrence risk Decreased; almost no recurrence rate[6] with use of folic acid supplementation and fortification.

Obstetric management In cases of spina bifida aperta, especially with a defect of the skin, a Cesarean section is preferable to protect the spinal cord and nerves and prevent infection.

Neurosurgical management

Spina bifida aperta In cases with a defect of normal skin tissue, immediate closure of spina bifida after birth reduces spinal infection. Spinal cord reconstruction is the most important part of the operation. Miniature Ommaya reservoir placement and a subsequent ventriculoperitoneal shunt are required for hydrocephalus (see Chapter 5). For symptomatic Chiari malformation, posterior fossa decompressive craniectomy and/or tonsillectomy is performed.

Spina bifida occulta The aim of surgical treatment is for decompression of the spinal cord and cutting off tethering to the spinal cord (Figures 6.22 and 6.23).

Cranium bifidum (Figures 6.24–6.32)

Prevalence Anencephaly, 0.29/1000 births[1]; overall neural tube defect (NTD), 0.58–1.17/1000 births[2,4,5]. Many authors have reported a remarkable reduction in prevalence of NTDs after using folic acid supplementation and fortification[1,2,4,5], although some have reported no decline of anencephaly rate[3].

Definition As in spina bifida, cranium bifidum has been classified into four types of encephaloschisis (including anencephaly and exencephaly), meningocele, encephalomeningocele, encephalocystocele and cranium bifidum occultum. Encephalocele occurs in the occipital region in 70–80% of cases. Acrania, exencephaly and anencephaly are not independent anomalies. It is considered that dysraphia (absent cranial vault, acrania) occurs at a very early stage and disintegration of the exposed brain (exencephaly) during the fetal period results in anencephaly[7].

Etiology Multifactorial inheritance, single mutant genes, specific teratogens (valproic acid), maternal diabetes and environmental factors. Predominant in females.

Pathogenesis Failure of anterior neural tube closure or a restricted disorder of neurulation.

Associated anomalies Open spina bifida (iniencephaly), Chiari type III malformation, bilateral renal cystic dysplasia and postaxial polydactyly with occipital cephalocele (Meckel–Gruber syndrome), hydrocephalus and polyhydramnios.

Prenatal diagnosis Figures 6.24–6.26 and 6.29; neonatal appearance, Figures 6.30 and 6.31.

Differential diagnosis Amniotic band syndrome (Figures 6.27 and 6.28, cranial destruction secondary to an amniotic band, similar appearance but different pathogenesis from acrania/excencephaly).

Prognosis Anencephaly is a uniformly lethal anomaly. Other types of cranium bifidum and various neurological deficits may occur, depending on types and degree.

Recurrence risk There used to be high recurrence risk of 5–13%; however, this has recently declined as described for spina bifida.

Obstetric management Termination of pregnancy can be offered in cases with anencephaly.

Neurosurgical management For other types of cranium bifidum, surgery aims to achieve transposition of cerebral tissue into the intracranial cavity (Figure 6.32). Ventriculoperitoneal shunt for hydrocephalus.

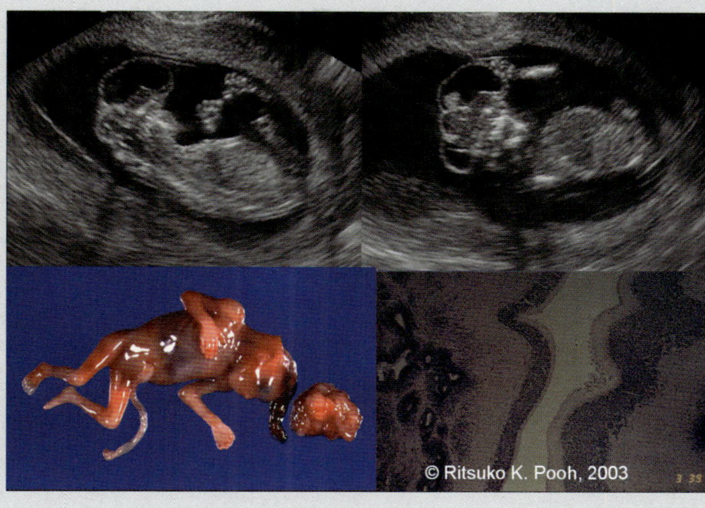

Figure 6.24 Acrania at 12 weeks of gestation. Upper, ultrasound sagittal and coronal images. The irregular surface of enlarged ventricles is demonstrated. Lower left, external appearance of the aborted fetus. Lower right, histology confirmed premature brain tissue

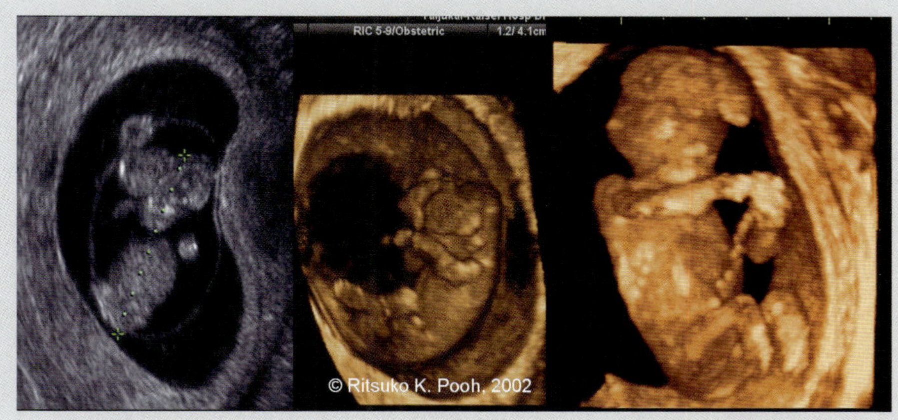

Figure 6.25 Acrania at 10 and 14 weeks of gestation. Left, ultrasound coronal image at 10 weeks. Note the normal appearance of the amniotic membrane, which indicates this condition is not amniotic band syndrome. Middle, three-dimensional ultrasound image of the same fetus as in the left image. Right, another case of acrania at 14 weeks

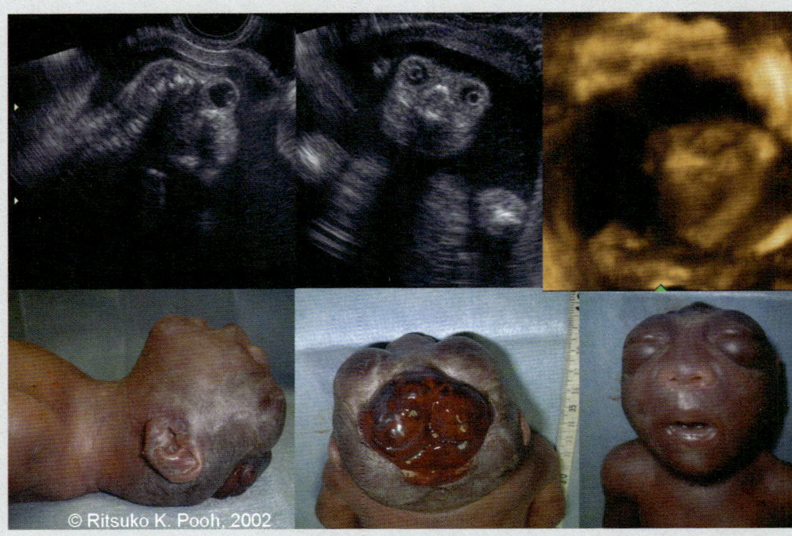

Figure 6.26 Anencephaly in middle gestation (same case as shown in Figure 6.25, left and middle). Upper left, ultrasound sagittal image at 23 weeks of gestation. Upper middle, ultrasound coronal image. Upper right, three-dimensional ultrasound image. Lower, external appearance of the stillborn fetus at 25 weeks of gestation. It is clear that excencephalic brain tissue is scattered in the amniotic space compared with this case at 10 weeks (Figure 6.25)

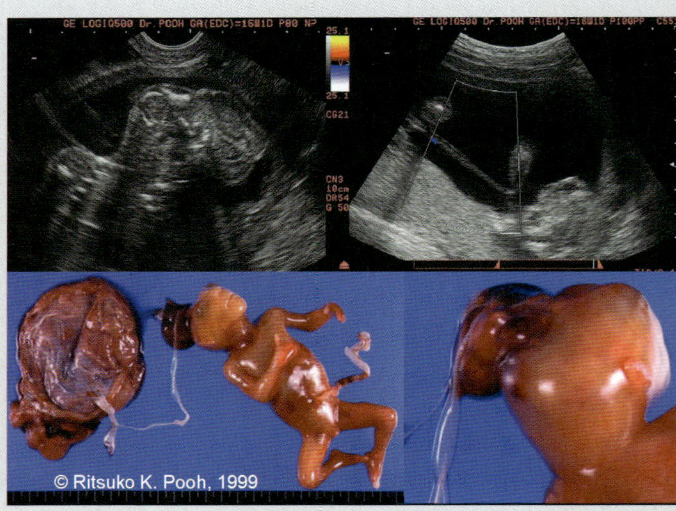

Figure 6.27 Amniotic band syndrome at 16 weeks of gestation. Upper left, exencephaly with an incomplete asymmetrical cranial defect. Upper right, amniotic band between placenta and exencephalic brain. Lower left, macroscopic appearance of the aborted fetus. Note the amniotic band between the placenta and brain. Lower right, magnified photograph of the head. This condition should be differentiated from encephaloschisis. Amniotic band syndrome has little risk of recurrence

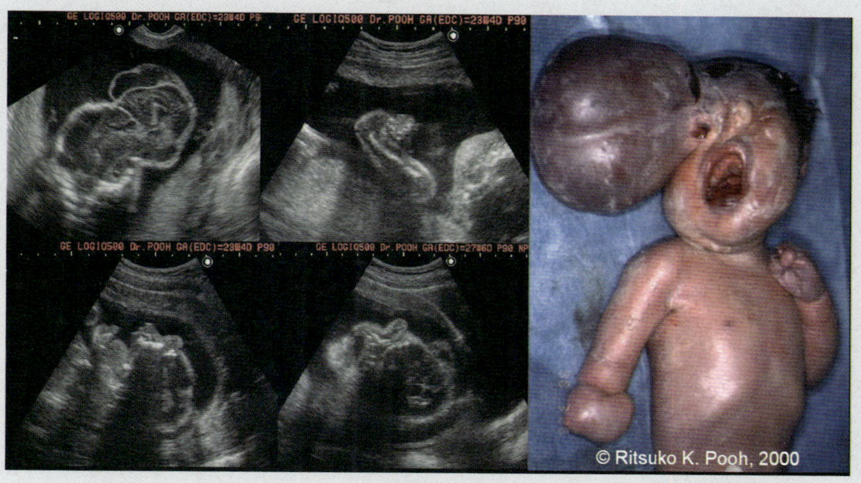

Figure 6.28 Amniotic band syndrome in middle gestation. Upper left, exencephaly with an incomplete asymmetrical cranial defect at 23 weeks of gestation. Upper middle, arm deformity. Lower left and middle, facial abnormality. The parents chose to continue the pregnancy. Right, photograph after birth at 33 weeks of gestation; the baby died one day postnatally. The exencephalic brain is covered with skin and amniotic membrane. Amniotic band syndrome should be differentiated from encephaloschisis

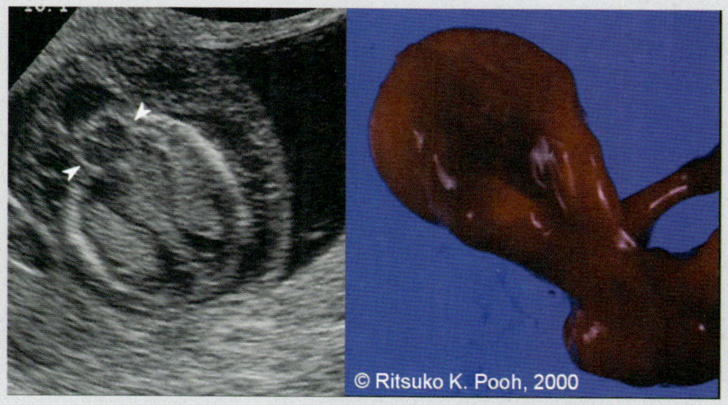

Figure 6.29 Encephalocele at 13 weeks of gestation. Left, brain tissue is protruding through the cranial defect (arrowheads). Right, photograph of the head of the same case after an artificial abortion

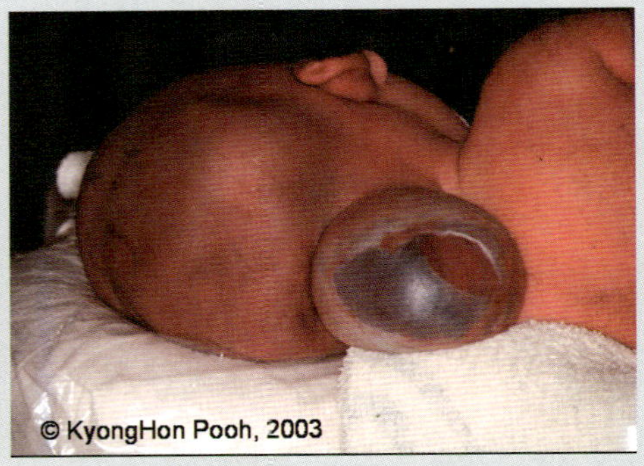

Figure 6.30 Occipital encephalomeningocele

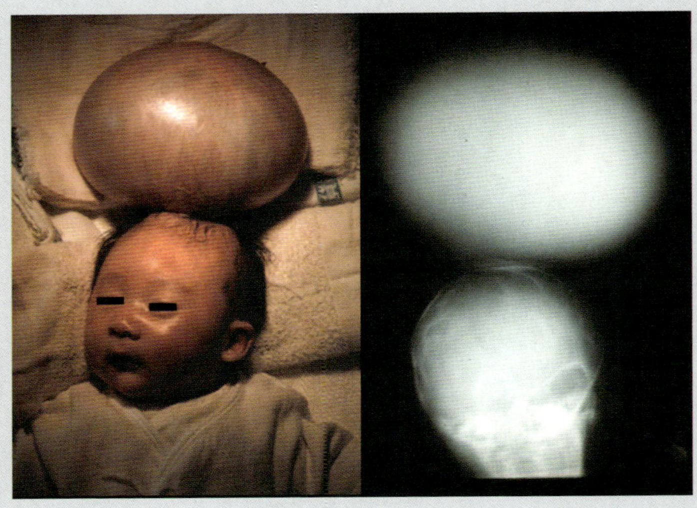

Figure 6.31 Parietal cephalocele. Left, photograph of head and huge parietal cephalocele. Right, a craniogram. The cyst, filled with a large amount of cerebrospinal fluid, was resected after birth. Image courtesy of Dr Y. Nakagawa

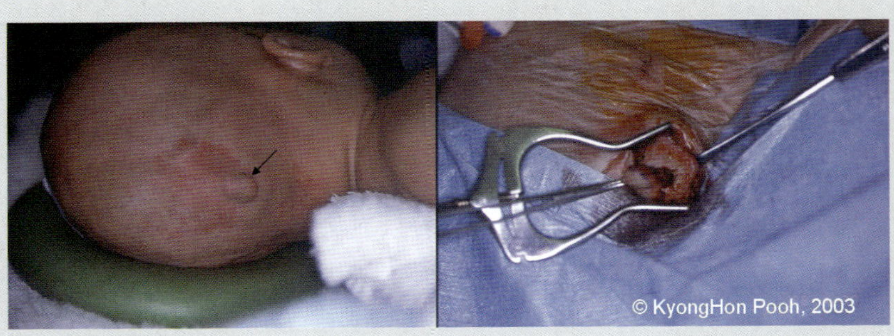

Figure 6.32 Cranium bifidum occultum. Left, photograph of the head. An occipital protrusion (arrow) penetrated into the intracranial space. Right, intraoperative photograph

CEREBRAL ANOMALIES

These include disorders of prosencephalic development and neuronal migration.

Holoprosencephaly (Figures 6.33–6.38)

Incidence 1 in 15 000–20 000 live births; however, initial incidence may be more than 60-fold greater in aborted human embryos[8,9].

Classification Holoprosencephalies (Figure 6.33) are classified into three varieties[10]:

(1) *Alobar type* A single-sphered cerebral structure with a single common ventricle, posterior large cyst of third ventricle (dorsal sac), absence of olfactory bulbs and tracts and a single optic nerve;

(2) *Semilobar type* With formation of a posterior portion of the interhemispheric fissure;

(3) *Lobar type* With formation of the interhemispheric fissure anteriorly and posteriorly but not in the mid-hemispheric region. The fusion of the fornices is seen[11].

Etiology 75% of cases of holoprosencephaly have a normal karyotype, but chromosomes 2, 3, 7, 13, 18 and 21 have been implicated in holoprosencephaly[10]. In particular, trisomy 13 has most commonly been observed. Autosomal dominant transmission is rare.

Pathogenesis Failure of cleavage of the prosencephalon and diencephalon during early first trimester (5–6 weeks) results in holoprosencephaly.

Associated anomalies Facial abnormalities such as cyclopia, ethmocephaly, cebocephaly, flat nose, cleft lip and palate are invariably associated with holoprosencephaly. Extracerebral abnormalities are also invariably associated, such as renal cysts/dysplasia, omphalocele, cardiac disease and or myelomeningocele.

Prenatal diagnosis Figures 6.34–6.36; a neonatal MRI and macroscopic appearance are shown in Figures 6.37 and 6.38.

Differential diagnosis Hydrocephalus, hydranencephaly.

Prognosis Extremely poor in alobar holoprosencephaly. Uncertain in lobar type. Various but poor in semilobar type.

Recurrence risk 6%[12], but much lower in sporadic or trisomy cases, much higher in genetic cases.

Management Chromosomal evaluation is offered.

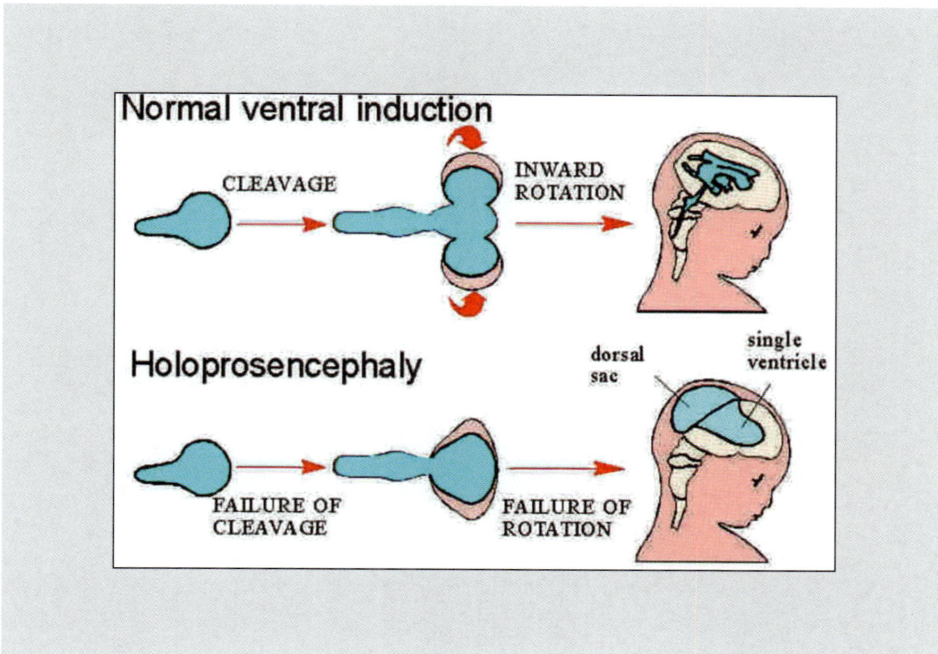

Figure 6.33 Normal and abnormal brain development leading to holoprosencephaly. Failure of sagittal cleavage of the telencephalon that results in the presence of a midline single ventricle with variable degrees of separation. Schema courtesy of Dr P. Jeanty, www.TheFetus.net, with permission

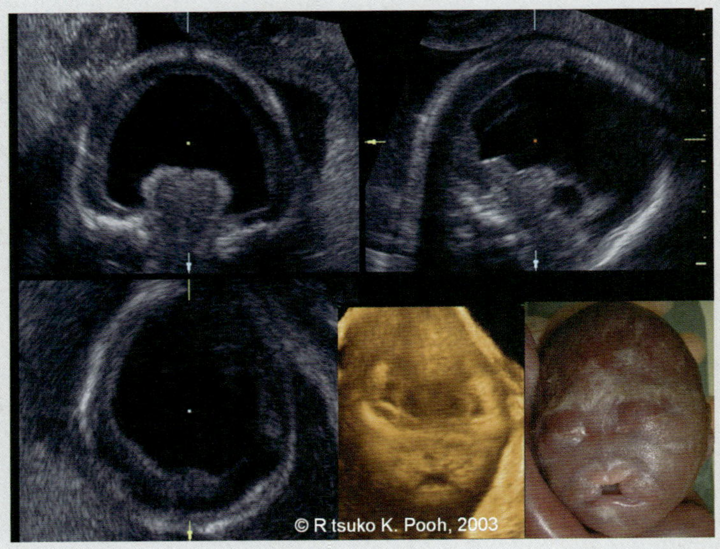

Figure 6.34 Alobar holoprosencephaly at 20 weeks of gestation. Three orthogonal images of intracranial structure show a complete single ventricle within a single-sphered cerebral structure. Lower right, three-dimensional ultrasound image of the fetal face and the face of the aborted fetus at 21 weeks of gestation. A flat nose with median cleft lip/palate can be seen. Normal karyotype

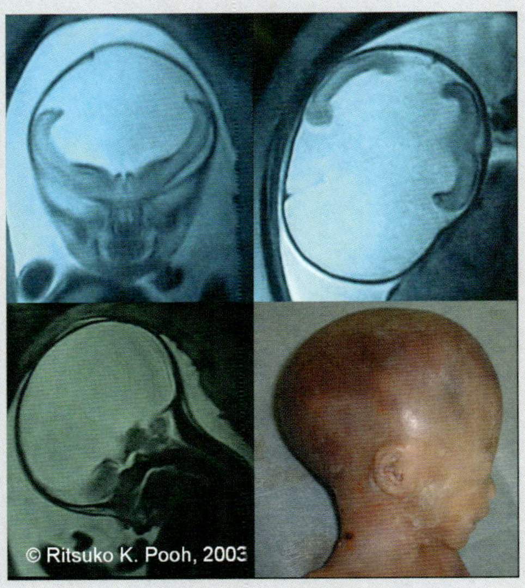

Figure 6.35 Fetal magnetic resonance (MR) images and macroscopic photograph of alobar holoprosencephaly. Upper, coronal and axial MR images. Lower left, sagittal MR image. Hydrocephalus is present in this case. Bilateral remnant of cerebral tissue is visible. Lower right, external appearance of the large head after birth. Normal karyotype

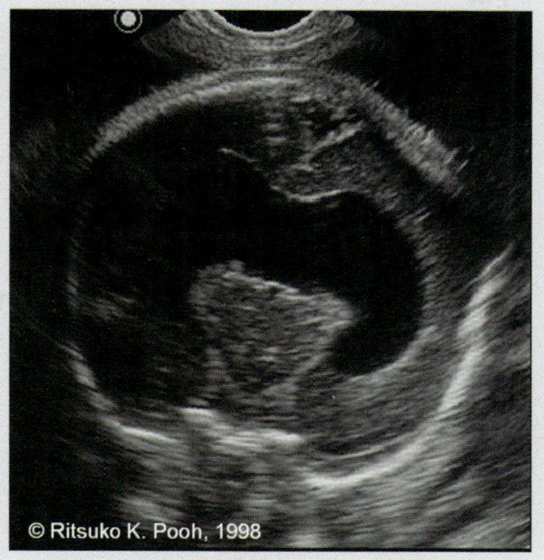

Figure 6.36 Fetal ultrasound image of semilobar holoprosencephaly at 28 weeks of gestation

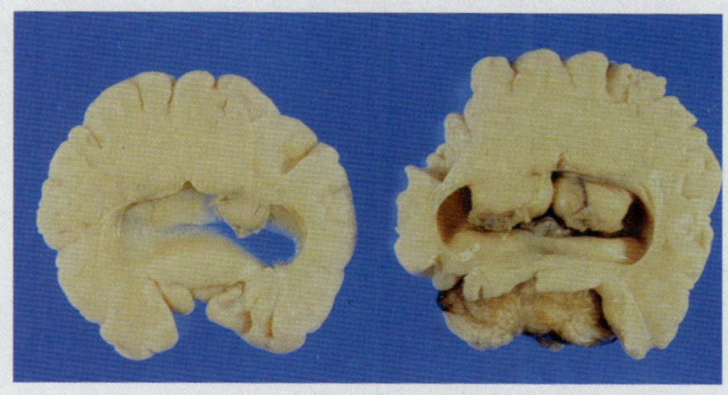

Figure 6.38 Macroscopic appearance of semilobar holoprosencephaly. Photograph courtesy of Dr Y. Nakagawa

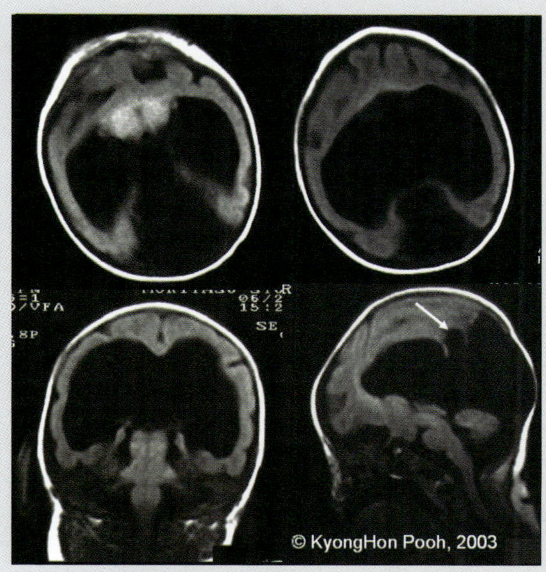

Figure 6.37 Postnatal magnetic resonance (MR) images of semilobar holoprosencephaly. Upper, MR axial images. A fused ventricle is demonstrated. Lower left, coronal image. Lower right, sagittal image. The white arrow indicates the dorsal sac. The cerebellum and brainstem are well developed. Hydrocephalus is also present

Agenesis, partial agenesis and hypogenesis of the corpus callosum (Figures 6.39–6.46)

Prevalence Uncertain, but 3–7/1000 in the general population is estimated.

Definition Absence of the corpus callosum (Figures 6.39 and 6.40), which may be divided into (complete) agenesis, partial agenesis or hypogenesis of the corpus callosum.

(1) *Complete agenesis* Complete absence of the corpus callosum;

(2) *Partial agenesis (hypogenesis)* Absence of splenium or posterior portion in various degrees.

Etiology Chromosomal aberration in 20% of affected cases, such as trisomy 18, 8 and 13. Autosomal dominant, autosomal recessive, X-linked recessive, part of the Mendelian syndrome such as Walker–Warburg syndrome, and X-linked dominant such as Aicardi's syndrome.

Pathogenesis Uncertain, but callosal formation may be associated with migration disorder.

Associated anomalies Colpocephaly (ventriculomegaly with disproportionate enlargement of trigones, occipital horns and temporal horns, not hydrocephaly), superior elongation of the third ventricle, interhemispheric cyst, lipoma of the corpus callosum.

Prenatal diagnosis Figures 6.41–6.45; neonatal MRI, Figure 6.46.

Diagnosis As the corpus callosum is depicted after 17 or 18 weeks of gestation by ultrasound, it is impossible to diagnose agenesis of the corpus callosum prior to this age[13].

Prognosis Various. Depends on associated anomalies. Most cases with isolated agenesis of the corpus callosum without other abnormalities are asymptomatic and prognosis is good. Complete agenesis has a worse prognosis than partial agenesis[14]. Epilepsy, intellectual impairment or psychiatric disorder[15] may occur later on.

Recurrence risk Depends on etiology. Chromosomal 1%; autosomal recessive 25%; X-linked recessive male 50%.

Management Standard obstetric care. Chromosomal evaluation should be offered. In cases with an interhemispheric cyst, postnatal fenestration or a shunt procedure may be performed.

Absent septum pellucidum and septo-optic dysplasia (Figure 6.47)

Incidence Unknown, rare.

Definition

(1) *Absent septum pellucidum* Absence of the septum pellucidum with or without associated anomalies. The septum pellucidum can be destroyed by concomitant hydrocephalus or by contiguous ischemic lesions such as porencephaly. An isolated absent septum pellucidum[16] exists but is rare.

(2) *Septo-optic dysplasia* Absence of the septum pellucidum and unilateral or bilateral hypoplasia of the optic nerve.

Synonyms de Morsier syndrome (septo-optic dysplasia).

Etiology Maternal drug (multidrug, valproic acid[17], cocaine[18]), autosomal recessive, *HESX1* homeodomain gene mutation[19].

Pathogenesis May occur as a vascular disruption sequence, with other prosencephalic or neuronal migration disorders.

Associated anomalies Schizencephaly, gyral abnormalities, heterotopias, hypotelorism, ventriculomegaly, communicating lateral ventricles, bilateral cleft lip and palate, hypopituitarism.

Prenatal diagnosis Figure 6.47.

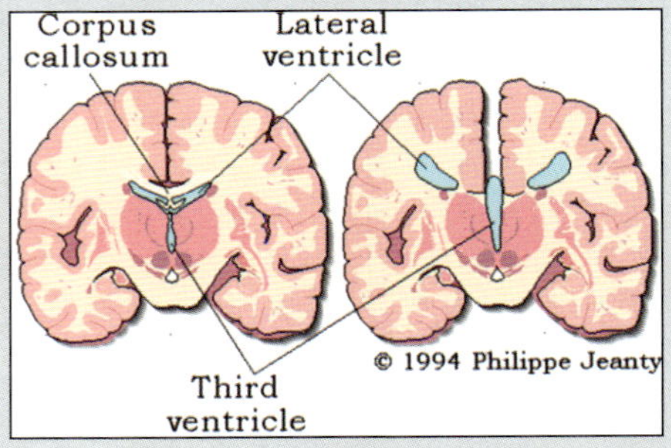

Figure 6.39 Schematic representations of a normal brain (left) and agenesis of the corpus callosum (right). In the absence of the corpus callosum, the lateral ventricles are set apart, and the third ventricle is displaced upwards. Schema courtesy of Dr P. Jeanty, www.TheFetus.net, with permission

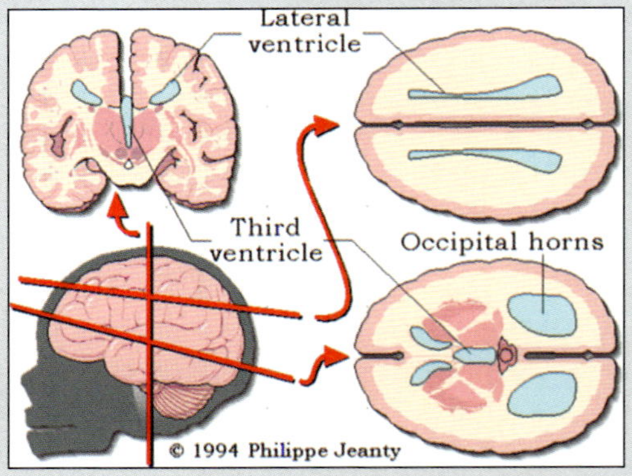

Figure 6.40 Schematic diagram of agenesis of the corpus callosum without an interhemispheric cyst. A coronal view (top left) shows that the lateral ventricles point superiorly. At the superior scan level (top right), both walls of the lateral ventricles are identified where only periventricular lines are normally present. The lower section (bottom right) shows dilatation of the occipital horns and separation of the frontal horns. The third ventricle may or may not be dilated. Diagram courtesy of Dr P. Jeanty, www.TheFetus.net, with permission

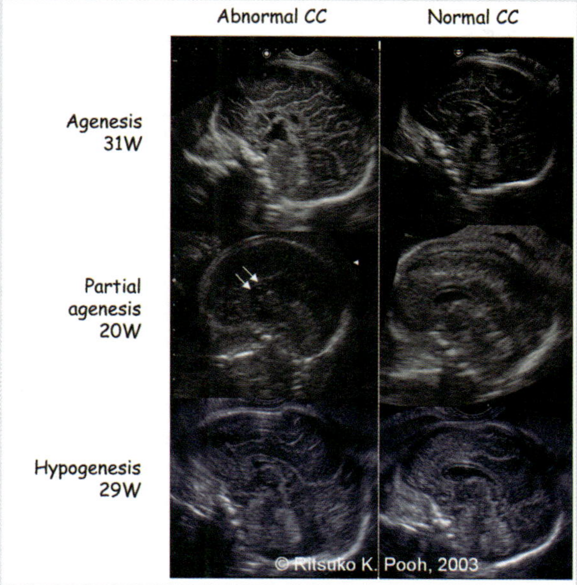

Figure 6.41 Agenesis, partial agenesis and hypogenesis of the corpus callosum (CC). All images are transvaginal median (mid-sagittal) images. Right images are normal images of the corpus callosum at the same gestational age as each left image

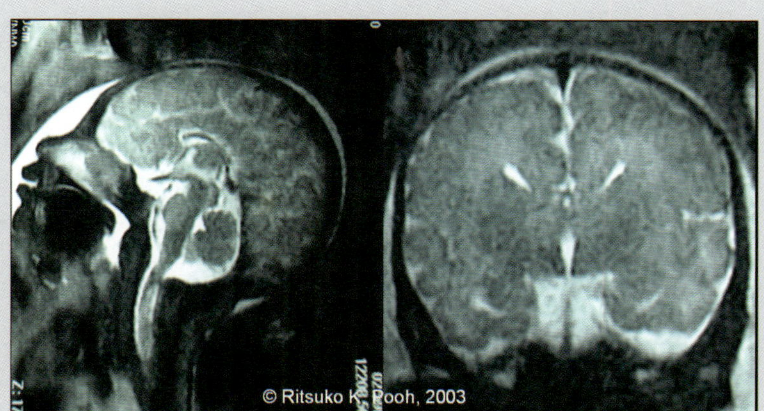

Figure 6.42 Fetal magnetic resonance images of hypogenesis of the corpus callosum at 34 weeks of gestation. (same case as shown in Figure 6.41, lower case). Sagittal and coronal images. In the sagittal image (left), the thin corpus callosum with obliterated cavum septum pellucidum is demonstrated. In the coronal section (right), the abnormal angle of the anterior horns of the lateral ventricles are depicted. No ventriculomegaly was present

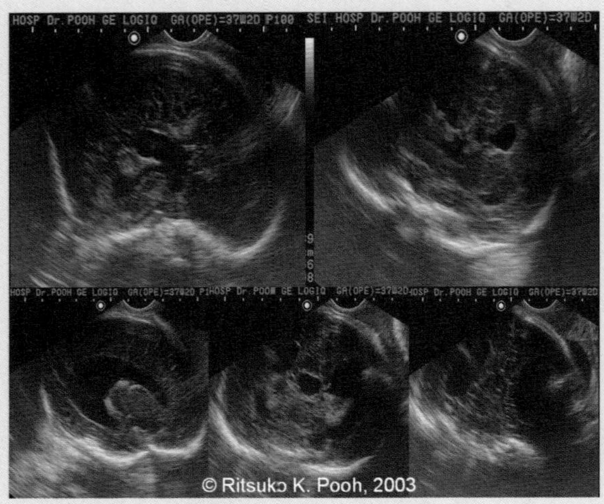

Figure 6.43 Fetal ultrasound images of hypogenesis of the corpus callosum at 37 weeks of gestation. The corpus callosum is thin and hypogenetic. Mild bilateral ventriculomegaly is present and typical colpocephaly is demonstrated in the lower left figure

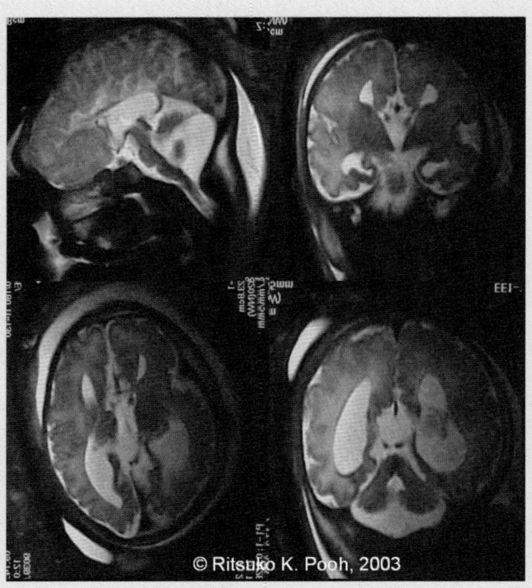

Figure 6.44 Fetal magnetic resonance images of hypogenesis of the corpus callosum with cerebellar hypoplasia (same case as shown in Figure 6.43). The corpus callosum is thin and hypogenetic. Cerebellar hypoplasia and an atrophic brainstem are demonstrated. Chromosomal abberation (partial trisomy/monosomy) was confirmed in this case. The baby died after several months in a vegetative state

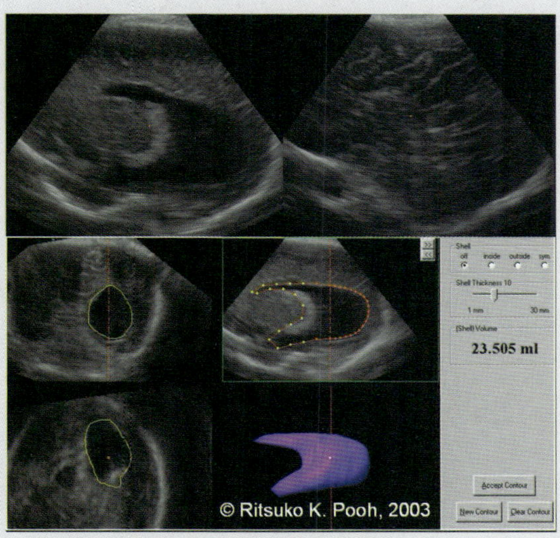

Figure 6.45 Colpocephaly associated with agenesis of the corpus callosum. Upper left, parasagittal section ultrasound image. Disproportionate enlargement of trigone and occipital horns of the lateral ventricle because of failure of development of the splenium of the corpus callosum and the calcarine fissure. Upper right, median section ultrasound image. No depiction of the corpus callosum and cingulate sulcus. Lower, three orthogonal views and a volume extraction image

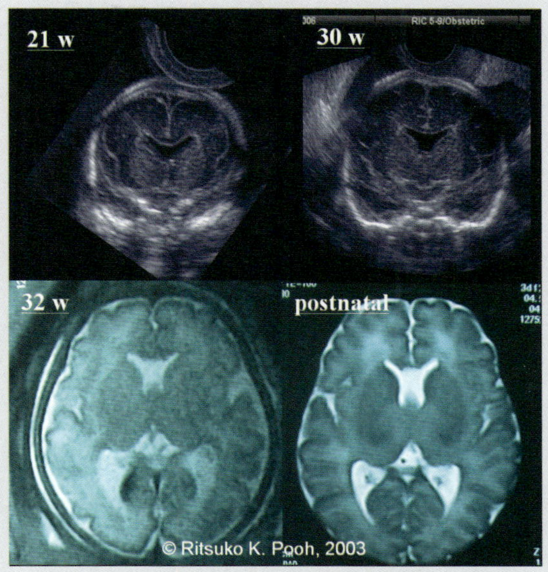

Figure 6.47 Isolated absent septum pellucidum. An absent septum pellucidum is mostly complicated by other CNS abnormalities and an isolated absent septum pellucidum is rare. This case has been carefully checked after birth by a pediatric neurologist and no neurological deficit has been found for 1 year after birth

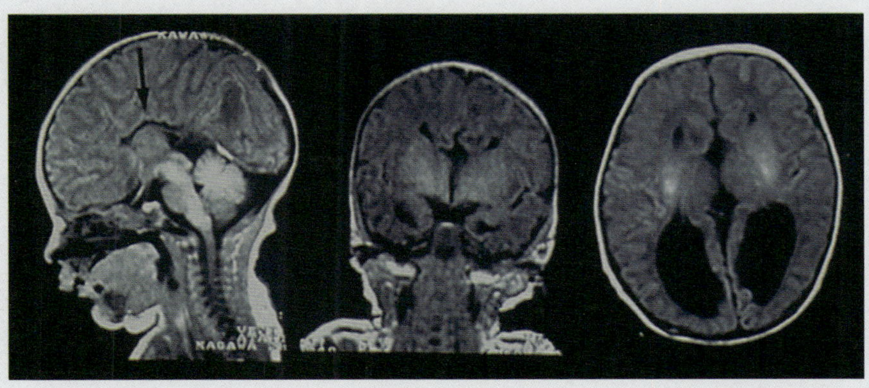

Figure 6.46 Agenesis of the corpus callosum (arrow); postnatal magnetic resonance images. Left, sagittal image. Note radiated sulci formation. Middle, coronal image. Note bull horn appearance of anterior horns of lateral ventricles. Right, axial image. Colpocephaly is seen. Images courtesy of Dr S. Endo

Differential diagnosis Dysgenesis of the corpus callosum, lobar holoprosencephaly.

Prognosis Depends on associated anomalies. Variable degree of mental deficiency and multiple endocrine dysfunction. In cases with isolated absence of septum pellucidum, prognosis may be good.

Recurrence risk Unknown.

Management Confirmation of diagnosis after birth is important for genetic counselling. Endocrine dysfunction should be looked for and corrected. Shunt procedure in cases with progressive ventriculomegaly.

Lissencephaly (Figures 6.48–6.51)

Incidence Unknown, rare.

Definition Characterized by a lack of gyral development (Figure 6.48) and divided into two types:

(1) *Lissencephaly type I* A smooth surface of the brain. The cerebral wall is similar to that of an approximately 12-week-old fetus[20];
   (a) Isolated lissencephaly;
   (b) Miller–Dieker syndrome with additional craniofacial abnormalities, cardiac anomalies, genital anomalies, sacral dimple, creases and/or clinodactyly;

(2) *Lissencephaly type II* Cobblestone appearance;
   (a) Walker–Warburg syndrome with macrocephaly, congenital muscular dystrophy, cerebellar malformation and retinal malformation;
   (b) Fukuyama congenital muscular dystrophy with microcephaly and congenital muscular dystrophy.

Synonyms Agyria, pachygyria; Walker–Warburg syndrome was known as HARD±E syndrome (hydrocephalus, agyria, retinal dysplasia, with or without encephalocele).

Etiology Isolated lissencephaly is linked to chromosome 17p13.3 and chromosome Xq24-q24. Miller–Dieker syndrome is also linked to chromosome 17p13.3. Walker–Warburg syndrome is of autosomal recessive inheritance. Fukuyama congenital muscular dystrophy is linked to chromosome 9q31, fukutin[21].

Pathogenesis Defective neuronal migration with four, rather than six, layers in the cortex.

Associated anomalies Polyhydramnios, less fetal movement, colpocephaly, agenesis of the corpus callosum, Dandy–Walker malformation. In Miller–Dieker syndrome, micrognathia, flat nose, high forehead, low-set ears, cardiac anomalies and genital anomalies in the male are often observed. In Walker–Warburg syndrome, retinal and cerebellar malformation, and congenital muscular dystrophy are observed in all cases.

Prenatal diagnosis Figure 6.49; neonatal MRI and macroscopic appearance are shown in Figures 6.50 and 6.51. Prenatal diagnosis[22–25] of lissencephaly without previous history of an affected child probably cannot be reliably made until 26–28 weeks' gestation[7].

Prognosis Type I: hypotonia, paucity of movements, feeding disturbance, seizures. The prognosis is poor and death occurs. Type II: severe seizures, mental disorders, severe muscle disease with hypotonia. Death in the first year is common.

Recurrence risk Depends on etiology.

Management Karyotyping is recommended to detect the chromosomal defect. Standard obstetric care.

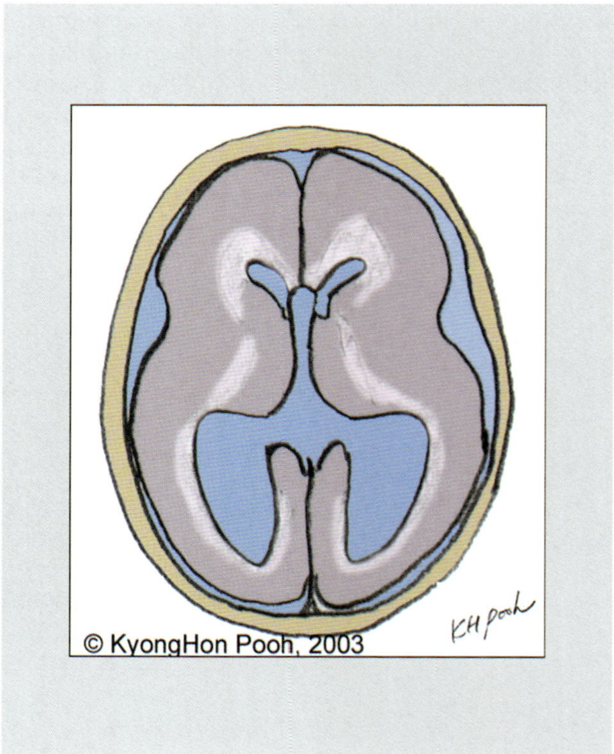

Figure 6.48 Schema of lissencephaly. Lissencephaly is characterized by no gyri formation and smooth brain with a shallow Sylvian fissure

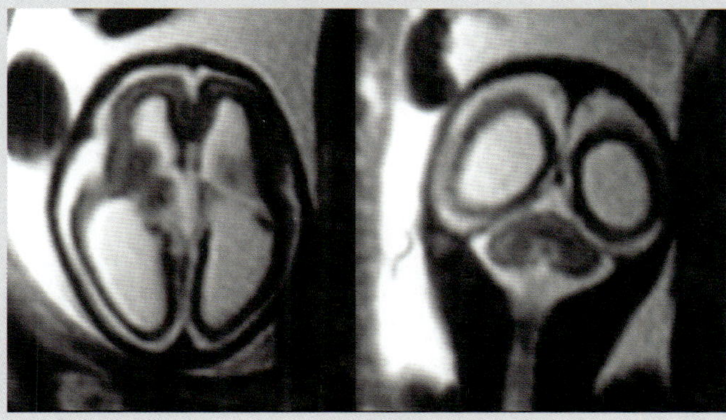

Figure 6.49 Fetal magnetic resonance image of type I lissencephaly at 30 weeks and 6 days of gestation. The cerebral cortex is thin and no gyral formation is observed. The fetus is one of dichorionic twins. The gyration of the other twin fetus was completely normal. Image courtesy of Dr H. Utsunomiya

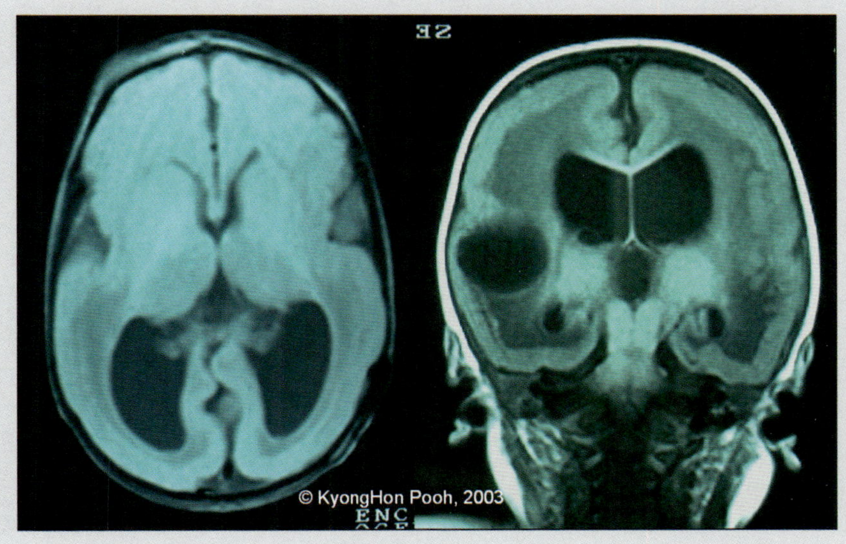

Figure 6.50 Magnetic resonance (MR) images of type I lissencephaly. Left, MR axial image. Neonatal lissencephaly. Smooth brain is demonstrated. There are a few gyral formations in the frontal area which indicates pachygyria in this part. Right, MR coronal image at 5 months in the same case. An intracranial cyst arose in the right lateral portion

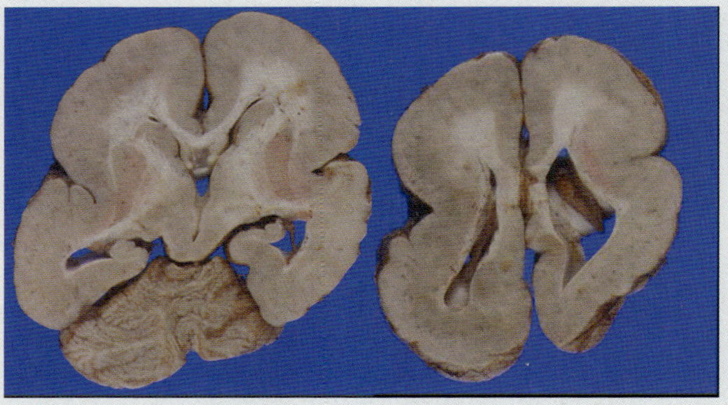

Figure 6.51 Microscopic photographs of type I lissencephaly. Left, smooth brain with a shallow Sylvian fissure is demonstrated. Note the cerebellar gyri and sulci are well formed. Photographs courtesy of Dr S. Endo

Schizencephaly (Figures 6.52 and 6.53)

Incidence Rare.

Definition A disorder characterized by congenital clefts in the cerebral mantle, lined by pia-ependyma, with communication between the subarachnoid space laterally and the ventricular system medially (Figure 6.52); 63% is unilateral and 37% bilateral; frontal region in 44% and frontoparietal 30%[20].

Etiology Uncertain. In certain familial cases, a point mutation in the homeobox gene, *EMX2* has been found[25,26]. Cytomegalovirus infection was also related in some cases[27].

Pathogenesis Neuronal migration disorder.

Associated anomalies Ventriculomegaly, microcephaly, polymicrogyria, gray-matter heterotopias, dysgenesis of the corpus callosum, absence of the septum pellucidum and optic nerve hypoplasia.

Differential diagnosis Porencephaly, arachnoid cyst or other intracranial cystic masses. MRI is useful in diagnosis of schizencephaly[28]. Neonatal schizencephaly is shown in Figure 6.53.

Prognosis Variable. Generally suffer from mental retardation, seizures, developmental delay and motor disturbances.

Recurrence risk Unknown.

Management Ventriculoperitoneal shunt for progressive hydrocephalus.

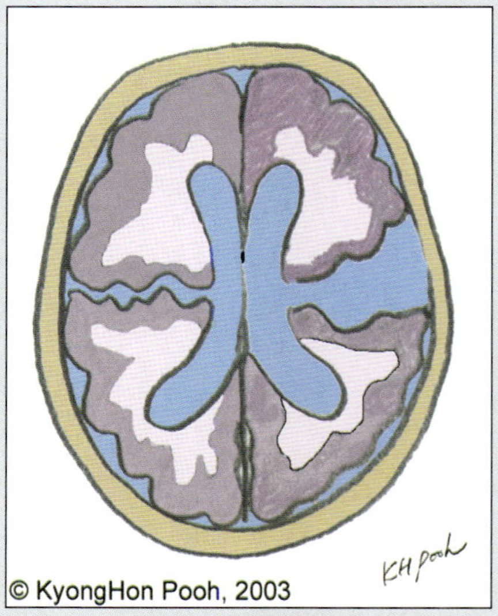

Figure 6.52 Schema of schizencephaly. Schizencephaly is characterized by clefts in the cerebral mantle, lined by pia-ependyma, with communication between the ventricles and the subarachnoid space; unilateral schizencephaly in 63% and bilateral in 37%. The cortical gray-matter lining of the cleft is important in differentiation from a destructive lesion such as porencephaly

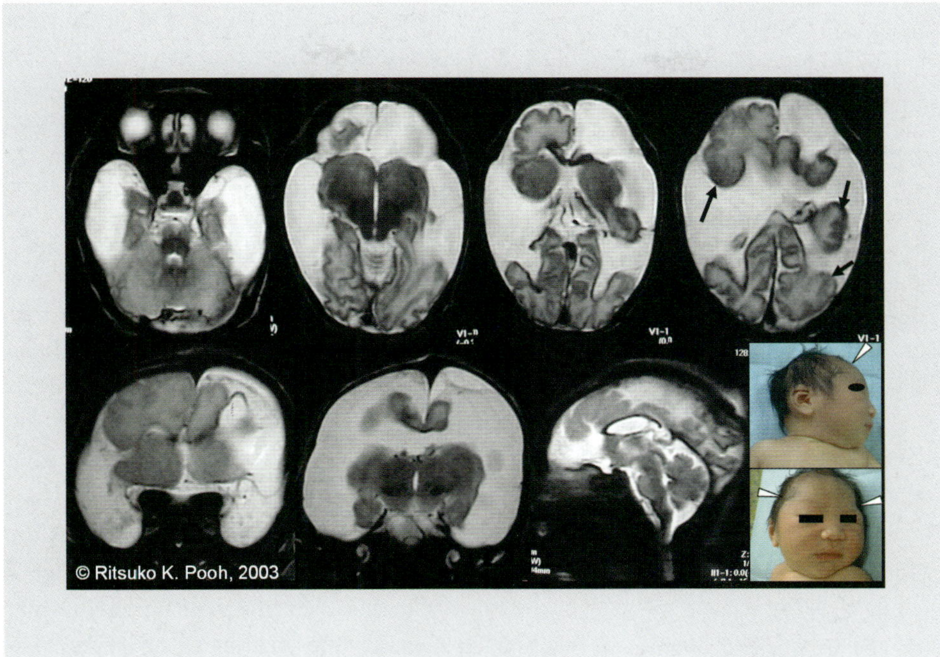

Figure 6.53 Magnetic resonance (MR) images of neonatal schizencephaly with porencephaly. Schizencephaly is a migrational disorder, characterized by unilateral or bilateral clefts in the cerebral mantle, lined by pia-ependyma, with communication between the ventricles and subarachnoid space. Gray matter of the cleft wall exhibits cortical dysplasia. MR axial images (upper) show bilateral schizencephaly and gray matter of the cleft wall is demonstrated. Lower, coronal and sagittal images. Porencephaly of the frontal lobe is also found in this case and a thin dysplastic corpus callosum is demonstrated. Posterior fossa development and the brainstem appear to be normal. No visits for check-ups were made during pregnancy; it was a home delivery. There was no growth retardation and no neonatal symptoms; however, a neonatal straight forehead and bilateral temple indentations (lower right, arrowheads) led to neonatal MR examination. Hydrocephaly was conspicuous 1 month after birth and a ventriculoperitoneal shunt was performed

POSTERIOR FOSSA ANOMALIES

Dandy–Walker malformation, Dandy–Walker variant and megacisterna magna (Figures 6.54–6.60)

Incidence Dandy–Walker malformation has an estimated prevalence of about 1/30 000 births, and is found in 4–12% of all cases of infantile hydrocephalus[29]. Incidence of Dandy–Walker variant and megacisterna magna is unknown.

Definition At present, the term Dandy–Walker complex[30] is used to indicate a spectrum of anomalies of the posterior fossa that are classified by axial CT scans as follows. Dandy–Walker malformation, Dandy–Walker variant and megacisterna magna seem to represent a continuum of developmental anomalies of the posterior fossa[29]:

(1) *(Classic) Dandy-Walker malformation* Cystic dilatation of the fourth ventricle, enlarged posterior fossa, elevated tentorium and complete or partial agenesis of the cerebellar vermis;

(2) *Dandy–Walker variant* Variable hypoplasia of the cerebellar vermis with or without enlargement of the posterior fossa;

(3) *Megacisterna magna* Enlarged cisterna magna with integrity of both cerebellar vermis and fourth ventricle.

Etiology Mendelian disorders such as Warburg's, chromosomal aberration such as 45,X, partial monosomy/trisomy, viral infections and diabetes.

Pathogenesis During the development of the fourth ventricular roof, a delay or total failure of the foramen of Magendie to open occurs, allowing a

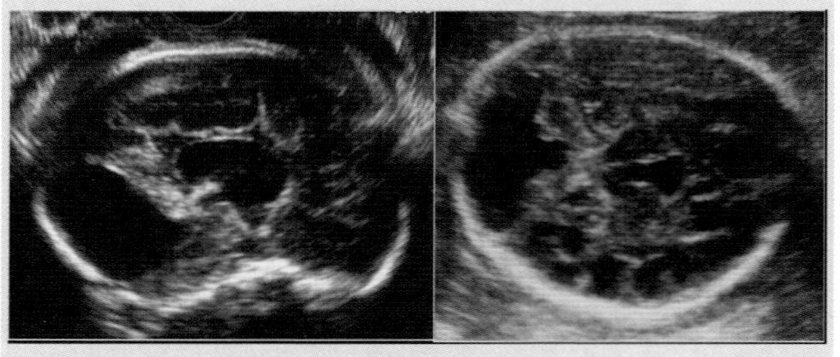

Figure 6.54 Dandy–Walker malformation (22 weeks of gestation) illustrated by a typical sagittal and axial image. A defect of the cerebellar vermis and an enlarged cisterna magna are demonstrated. Image courtesy of Dr V. D'Addario

build up of CSF and development of the cystic dilatation of the fourth ventricle. Despite the subsequent opening of the foramina of Luschka (usually patent in Dandy–Walker malformations), cystic dilatation of the fourth ventricle persists and CSF flow is impaired[10].

Associated anomalies of Dandy–Walker malformation Hydrocephalus and other midline anomalies, such as agenesis of the corpus callosum and holoprosencephaly and occipital encephalocele. Extracranial abnormalities such as congenital heart disease, neural tube defects and cleft lip/palate. A frequency of additional anomalies ranges between 50 and 70%.

Prenatal diagnosis Dandy–Walker malformation is shown in Figure 6.54, a Dandy–Walker variant in Figure 6.57 and megacisterna magna in Figures 6.58 and 6.59. To observe the agenesis of the cerebellar vermis, the axial cutting section is preferable. To observe the elevated tentorium, the sagittal section is preferable.

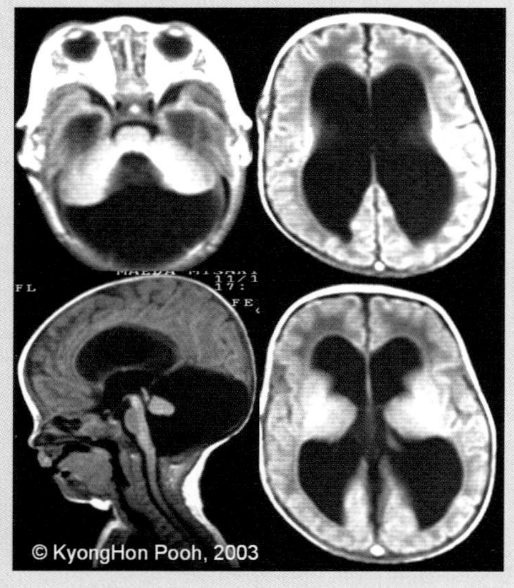

Figure 6.55 Postnatal magnetic resonance imaging of Dandy–Walker syndrome with hydrocephalus (1 day postnatally, before treatment). Upper left, axial section. Agenesis of the cerebellar vermis is demonstrated. Lower left, sagittal section. Note the posterior fossa cyst communicating with the IVth ventricle. Hydrocephalus is often present (upper/lower right)

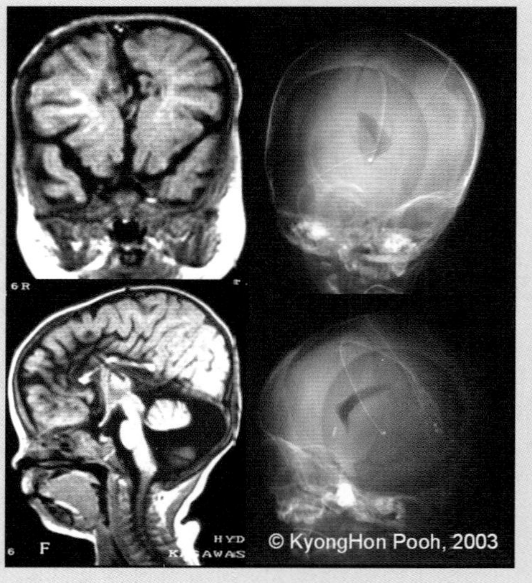

Figure 6.56 Post-treatment magnetic resonance image (MRI) and X-ray images of a Dandy-Walker case (same case as shown in Figure 6.55). Because of no communication between the supra- and infratentorial spaces, a supratentorial ventricular catheter and infratentorial cystic catheter were placed, and both catheters were connected to the abdominal catheter by a Y-connector

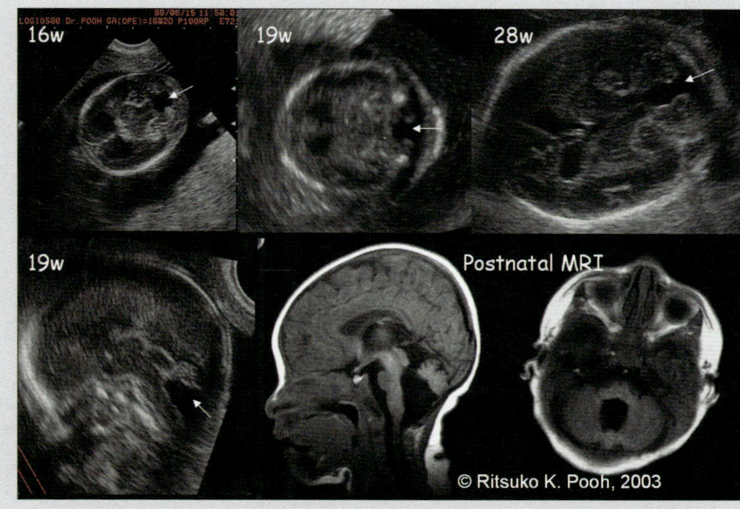

Figure 6.57 Dandy–Walker variant (from 16 weeks of gestation till newborn). Upper ultrasound axial sections at 16, 19 and 28 weeks. The sizes of the cerebellar and cisterna magna are normal, but the cerebellar vermis is not demonstrated and communication between the IVth ventricle and the cisterna magna is seen. Lower left, tranvaginal ultrasound sagittal image at 19 weeks. The cerebellum is floating in the posterior fossa. Lower middle and right, postnatal magnetic resonance image. Hypogenesis of the cerebellar vermis was confirmed. Normal development was seen at the age of 3 years

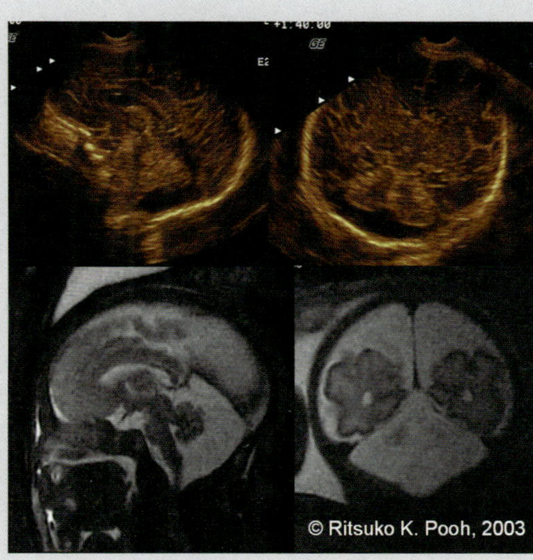

Figure 6.58 Fetal ultrasound/magnetic resonance (MR) images of megacisterna magna – fetal ultrasound sagittal/coronal sections (upper) and MR sagittal/coronal sections (lower). Cisterna magna seems to be large but no tentorial disproportion is seen. Cerebellar development has been normal

Differential diagnosis Infratentorial arachnoid cyst, other intracranial cystic tumors, hydrocephalus, cerebellar dysplasia (Figure 6.60).

Prognosis Progressive hydrocephalus; not observed in neonates but often progressive during the first month. In cases diagnosed *in utero* or in the neonatal period, outcome is generally unfavorable. Nearly 40% die, and 75% of survivors exhibit cognitive deficits[10]. Prognosis of the Dandy–Walker variant is good. Clinical significance of megacisterna magna is uncertain.

Recurrence risk Depends on etiology; generally 1–5% (Dandy–Walker malformation).

Management Cystoperitoneal shunt or cystoventriculoperitoneal shunt (Figures 6.55 and 6.56).

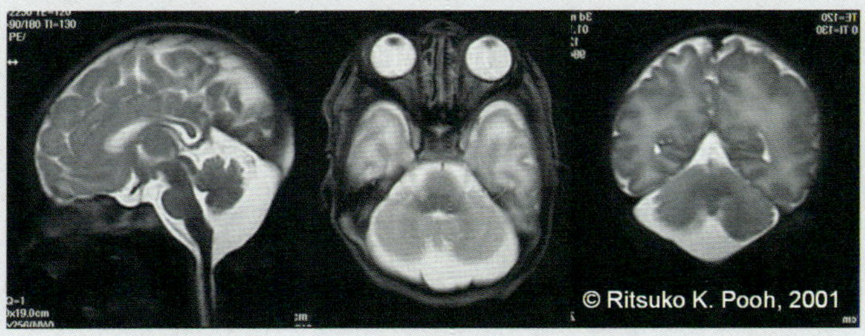

Figure 6.59 Neonatal magnetic resonance images (MRIs) of megacisterna magna (same case as shown in Figure 6.58). The large cisterna magna has spontaneously improved compared with the prenatal MRIs (Figure 6.58). Normal development was observed at the age of 2 years

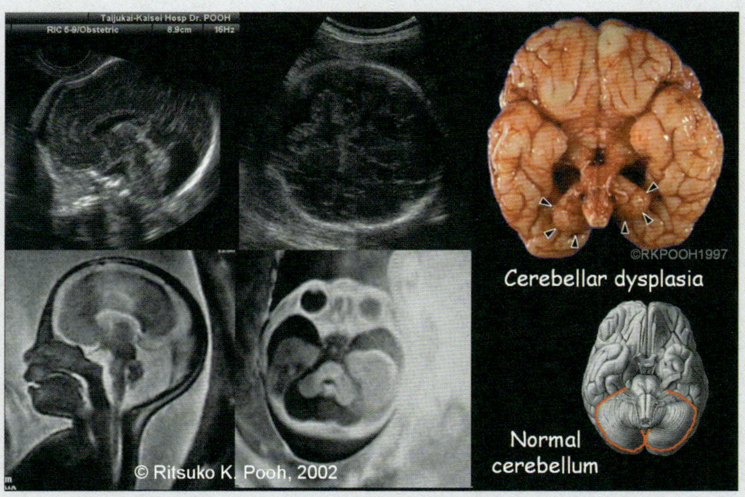

Figure 6.60 Cerebellar dysplasia. Differentiated diagnosis of the Dandy–Walker complex. Upper left, transvaginal median image of a small cerebellum within a normal-sized posterior fossa. Upper middle, transabdominal axial image. Lower left, fetal magnetic resonance sagittal image. Lower middle, magnetic resonance axial image. This case has the chromosomal aberration of trisomy 18. Upper right, macroscopic photograph of cerebellar dysplasia in another case of trisomy 18. Cerebellar dysplasia should be differentiated from the Dandy–Walker malformation, variant or megacisterna magna

Chiari malformation (Figures 6.61–6.69)

Prevalence Depends on prevalence of spina bifida (Chiari type II malformation). Following a recent remarkable reduction of prevalence of NTDs after using folic acid supplementation and fortification, prevalence has declined (see 'Spina bifida' in this Chapter). Other types are rare.

Definition Chiari anomalies with cerebellar herniation in the spinal canal were classified into three types according to the contents of the herniated tissue. The contents of type I is a lip of cerebellum, of type II part of the cerebellum, fourth ventricle and medulla oblongata, pons, and of type III a large herniation of the posterior fossa. Thereafter, type IV with just cerebellar hypogenesis was added. However, this classification occasionally leads to confusion in neuroimaging diagnosis. Therefore, at present, the classification as below is advocated:

(1) *Type I* Herniation of the cerebellar tonsil only, not associated with myelomeningocele;
(2) *Type II* (Figures 6.61 and 6.62). Herniation of the cerebellar tonsil and brainstem. Medullary kink, tentorial dysplasia, associated with myelomeningocele;
(3) *Type III* Associated with cephalocele or cranio-cervical meningocele, in which the cerebellum and the brainstem are herniated;
(4) *Type IV* Associated with marked cerebellar hypogenesis and posterior fossa shrinking.

Synonyms Arnold–Chiari malformation.

Etiology Depends on the type. (See 'Spina bifida' and 'Cranium bifidum' in this Chapter.)

Pathogenesis

(1) Inferior displacement of the medulla and the fourth ventricle into the upper cervical canal;
(2) Elongation and thinning of the upper medulla and lower pons and persistence of the embryonic flexure of these structures;
(3) Inferior displacement of the lower cerebellum through the foramen magnum into the upper cervical region;
(4) A variety of bony defects of the foramen magnum, occiput and upper cervical vertebrae[10].

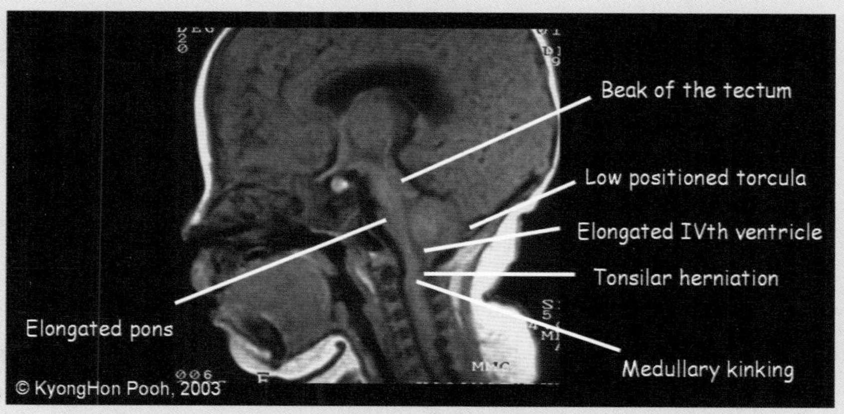

Figure 6.61 Magnetic resonance image of Chiari type II malformation. Anatomical characteristics of Chiari type II malformation (beak of the tectum, low-positioned torcula, elongated IVth ventricle, tonsillar herniation, medullary kinking and elongated pons) are shown in this picture. A chiari type II malformation is caused by the downward herniation of the posterior fossa contents probably due to cerebrospinal fluid leakage from open spina bifida

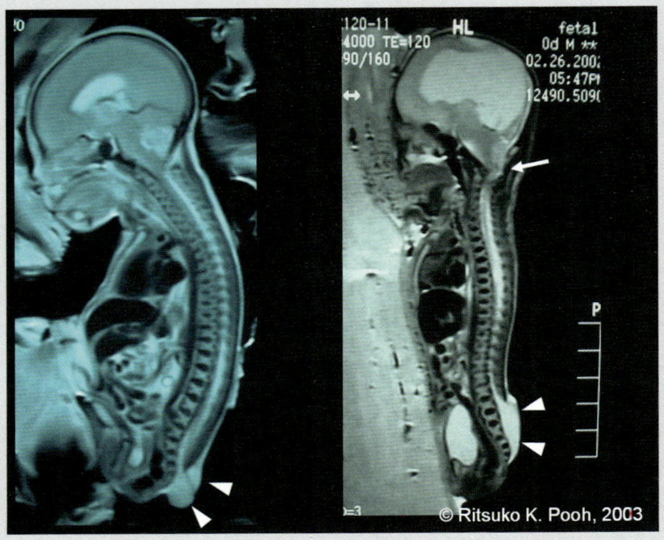

Figure 6.62 Magnetic resonance images of aborted fetuses at 20–21 weeks of gestation. Left, 20 weeks of gestation. Sacral myelomeningocele (arrowheads) and Chiari type II malformation are demonstrated. Right, 21 weeks of gestation. Lumbosacral myelomeningocele with Chiari type II malformation is seen. In this case, myelomeningocele is complicated by holoprosencephaly. Normal karyctype. A severe medullary kink (arrow) can be seen

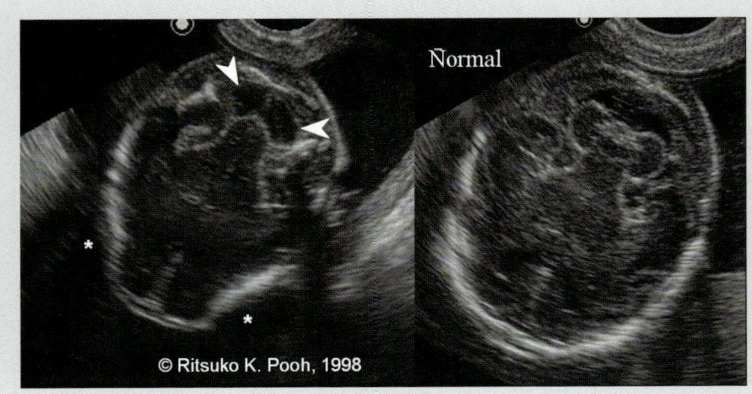

Figure 6.63 Chiari type II malformation at 19 weeks of gestation. Left, the ultrasound axial image shows a typical lemon sign (asterisks) and a typical banana sign (arrowheads). Right, comparative normal image in the same cutting section at the same gestation

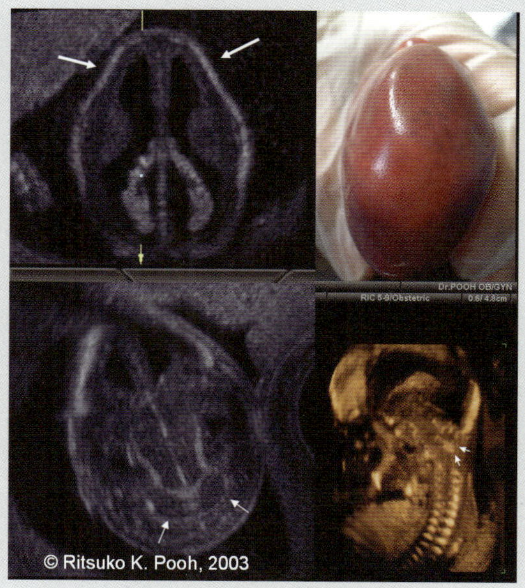

Figure 6.64 Chiari type II malformation at 16 weeks of gestation. Upper left, typical lemon sign (arrows). Upper right, external lemon-shaped head appearance of the aborted fetus. Lower left, typical banana sign (arrows). Lower right, three-dimensional reconstruction internal image of a Chiari type II malformation (arrows)

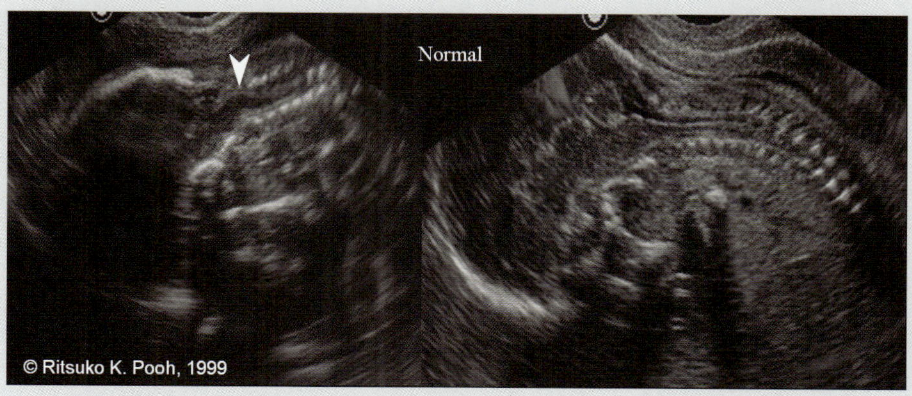

Figure 6.65 Medullary kink in a case of Chiari II malformation at 19 weeks of gestation. Left, medullary kink (arrowhead) associated with an obliterated cisterna magna is demonstrated. Right, comparative normal image in the same cutting section at the same gestation. The cisterna magna, cerebellum and medullospinal portion are clearly demonstrated

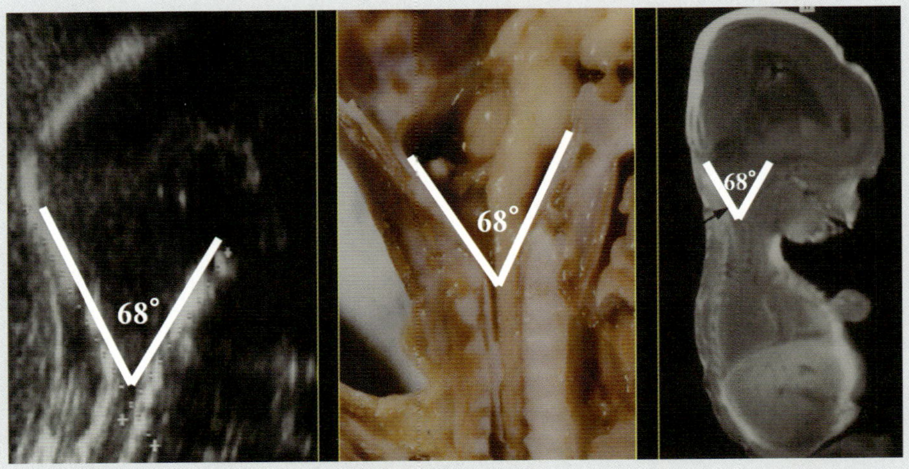

Figure 6.66 Clivus–supraocciput angle. Left, ultrasound sagittal image. Middle, macroscopic appearance. Right, magnetic resonance image. Measurement of the clivus–supraocciput angle in a 21-week-old fetus affected by Chiari malformation. The angle (68°) between the lines is lower than normal. Images courtesy of Dr V. D'Addario

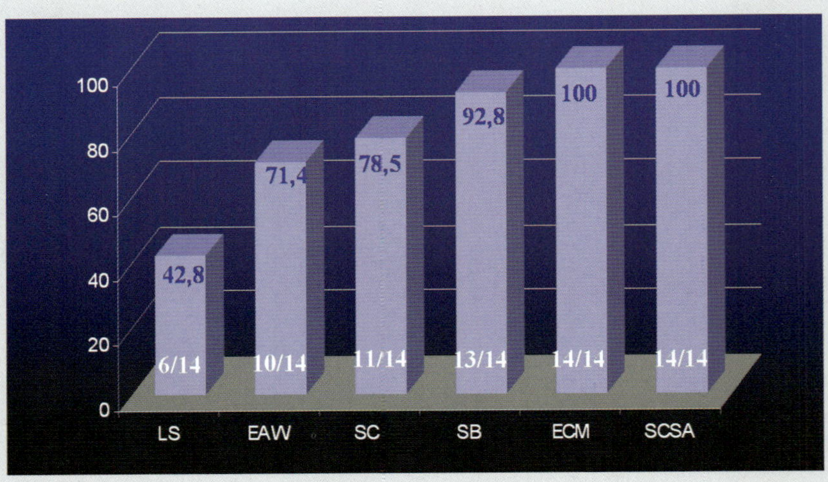

Figure 6.67 Features of a Chiari type II malformation. The evaluation of the posterior fossa and particularly the measurement of the clivus–supraocciput angle is a useful parameter to differentiate the various causes of fetal ventriculomegaly and particularly to recognize Chiari II malformation. LS, lemon sign; EAW, enlarged atrial width (> 12 mm); SC, small cerebellum (< 10°); SB, spina bifida; ECM, effaced cisterna magna; SCSA, small clivus–supraocciput angle (< 72°). Image courtesy of Dr V. D'Addario

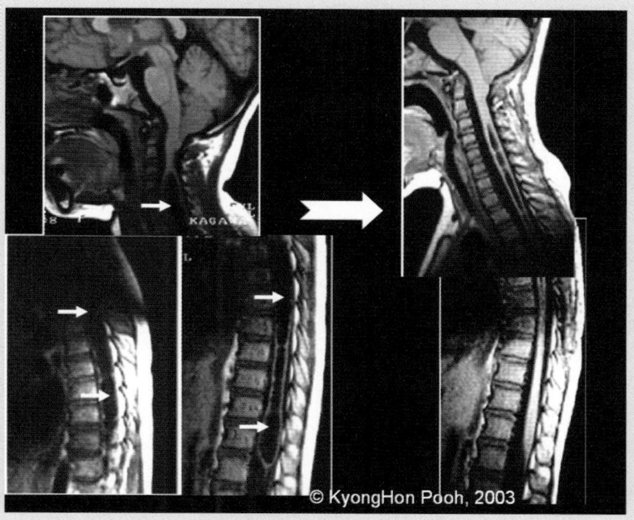

Figure 6.68 Chiari type I with syringohydromyelia in a 4-year-old female infant with onset of motor disturbance of the lower extremities. Left, tonsillar herniation and holocord syringohydromyelia (arrows) are demonstrated. Right, postoperative magnetic resonance image. The syrinx was markedly resolved and clinical symptoms disappeared after a syrinx–subarachnoid shunt

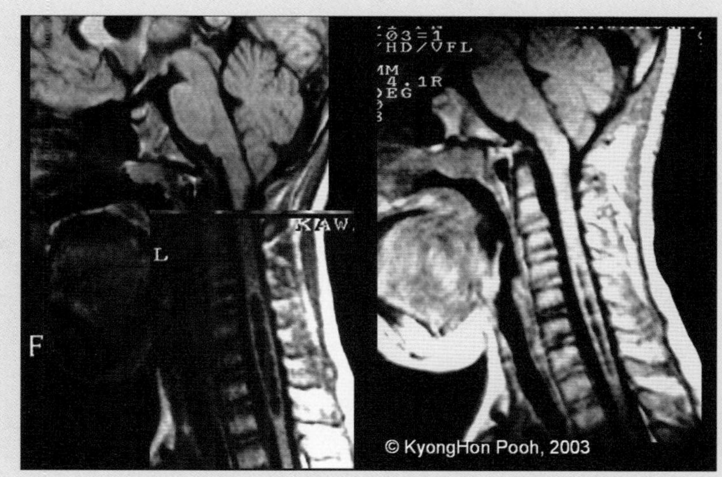

Figure 6.69 Chiari type I with syringohydromyelia in a 6-year-old male infant with onset of headache and dizziness. Left, mild tonsillar herniation and syringohydromyelia of the cervical spinal cord are demonstrated. Right, postoperative magnetic resonance image. The syrinx was resolved and clinical symptoms disappeared after foramen magnum decompression and C1 laminectomy

Associated anomalies Hydrocephalus caused by obstruction of fourth ventricular outflow or associated aqueductal stenosis. Myelomeningocele or myeloschisis (type II), cephalocele or craniocervical meningocele (type III), cerebellar hypogenesis (type IV) and syringohydromyelia (type I).

Prenatal diagnosis Prenatal ultrasound diagnosis by features: lemon sign which indicates deformity of the frontal bone, banana sign which indicates abnormal shape of the cerebellum without cisterna magna space (Figures 6.63 and 6.64), medullary kink (Figure 6.65) and small clivus–supraocciput angle (Figures 6.66 and 6.67)[31].

Differential diagnosis Craniosynostosis.

Prognosis Nearly every case of myelomeningocele is accompanied by a morphological Chiari II malformation. Many cases with Chiari II are asymptomatic. However, clinical features due to Chiari malformation, such as feeding disturbances, laryngeal stridor or apneic episode, are found in approximately 9–30% of cases. In cases with these clinical features, vital prognosis is often poor.

Recurrence risk Depends on type of Chiari malformation. Decreased according to decline of NTD recurrence rate by use of folic acid supplementation and fortification. (See 'Spina bifida' in this Chapter).

Neurosurgical management Neurosurgical decompression of foramen magnum for any types of Chiari malformation; syringo-subarachnoid shunt for Chiari type I (Figures 6.68 and 6.69).

Rhombencephalosynapsis (Figure 6.70)

Incidence Extremely rare.

Definition Characterized by dorsal fusion of the cerebellar hemispheres, an absence of the anterior vermis and a deficiency of the posterior vermis[32], fusion of dentate nuclei and superior cerebellar peduncles.

Etiology Molecular analysis of dorsalizing genes, such as *Lmx1a*, which regulate early developmental events at the pontomesencephalic junction, may reveal a mutation or mutations unique to rhombencephalosynapsis.

Pathogenesis This spectrum of anomalies is consistent with rhombencephalosynapsis and could be explained by an embryological defect of dorsal patterning that affects the 'isthmic organizer' at the mesencephalic–metencephalic border[33].

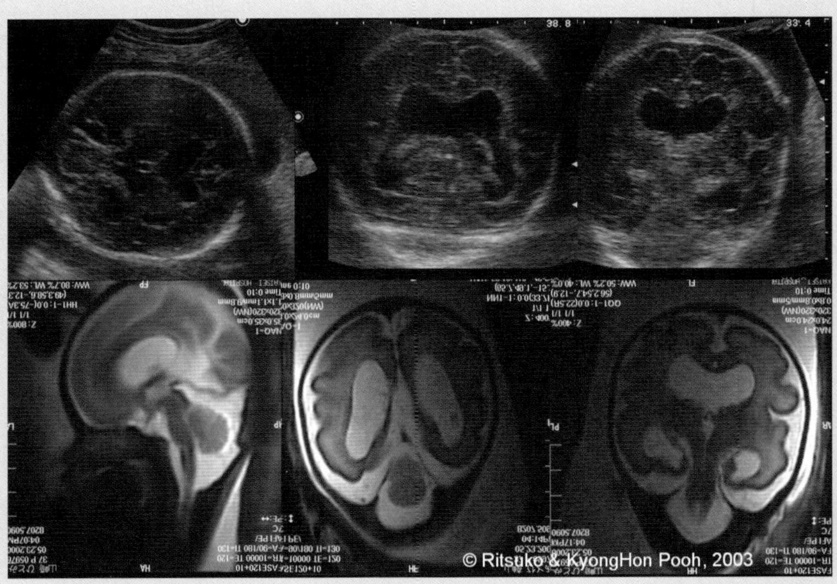

Figure 6.70 Fetal ultrasound and magnetic resonance images of rhombencephalosynapsis at 30 weeks of gestation. Upper, ultrasound images. Cerebellar fusion is seen in the axial section. Coronal sections show moderate ventriculomegaly and absent septum pellucidum. Lower, fetal magnetic resonance images

Associated anomalies Hydrocephalus, ventriculomegaly, additional supratentorial abnormalities, craniosynostosis, trigeminal anesthesia, alopecia.

Prenatal diagnosis Figure 6.70.

Differential diagnosis Cerebellar dysplasia, megacisterna magna and Chiari malformation.

Prognosis From mild truncal ataxia and normal cognitive abilities to severe cerebral palsy and mental retardation[34].

Recurrence risk Unknown.

Management Shunt procedure for infants with progressive hydrocephalus.

CRANIAL BONE ANOMALIES

Craniosynostosis (Figures 6.71–6.83)

Incidence Unknown.

Definition Premature closure of cranial suture, which may affect one or more cranial sutures. Simple sagittal synostosis is most common. Various cranial shapes depend on affected suture(s) (Figures 6.73–6.83).

(1) *Sagittal suture* Scaphocephaly or dolichocephaly;

(2) *Bilateral coronal suture* Brachycephaly;

(3) *Unilateral coronal suture* Anterior plagiocephaly;

(4) *Metopic suture* Trigonocephaly;

(5) *Lamboid suture* Acrocephaly;

(6) *Unilateral lamboid suture* Posterior plagiocephaly;

(7) *Coronal/lamboid/metopic or squamous/sagittal suture* Cloverleaf skull;

(8) *Total cranial sutures* Oxycephaly.

Syndromes

(1) *Crouzon syndrome* Acrocephaly, synostosis of coronal, sagittal and lamboid sutures; with ocular proptosis maxillary hypoplasia.

(2) *Apert syndrome* Brachycephaly, irregular synostosis, especially coronal suture; with midfacial hypoplasia, syndactyly, broad distal phalanx of thumb and big toe.

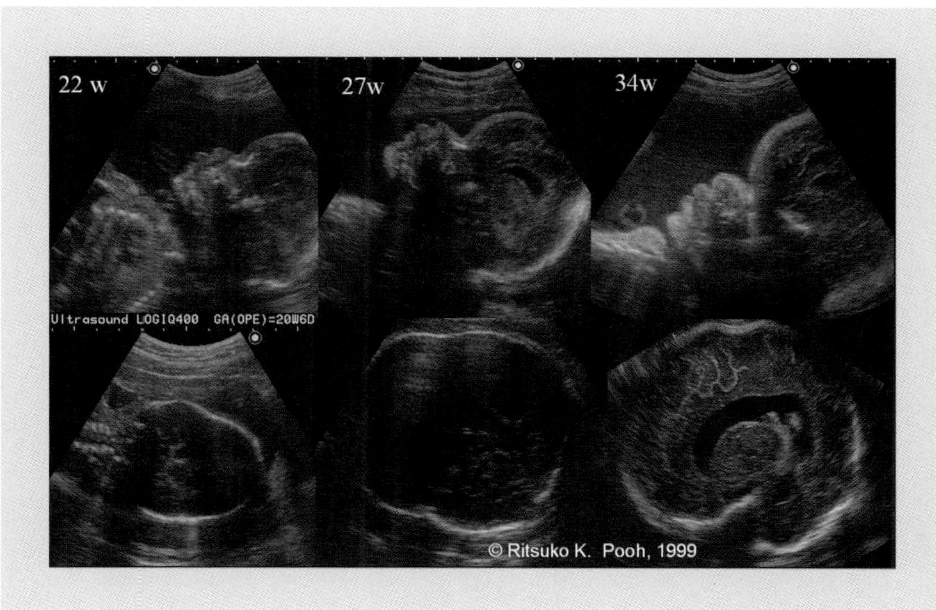

Figure 6.71 Prenatal craniofacial appearance of Apert syndrome (see Figures 6.74–6.76 for treatment of this case). Upper, longitudinal changing appearance of frontal bossing and low nasal bridge at 22, 27 and 34 weeks of gestation in a case of Apert syndrome. Lower left, irregular cranial shape at 20 weeks. Lower middle, cranial shape at 34 weeks. Note the bilateral indentation. Lower right, intracranial sagittal ultrasound image at 34 weeks. Mild ventriculomegaly is present

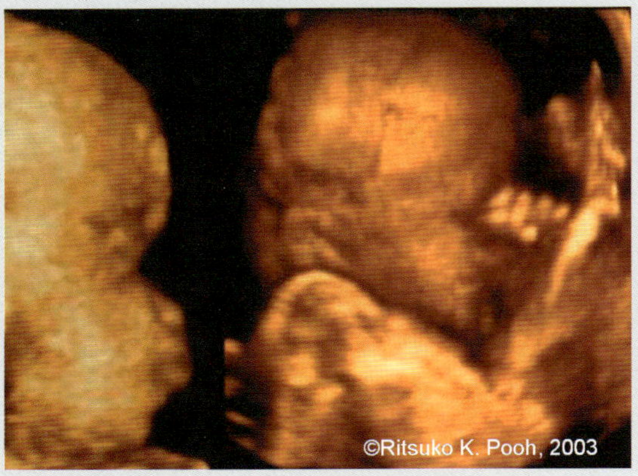

Figure 6.72 Three-dimensional ultrasound images of craniosynostosis with frontal bossing and low nasal bridge. Although the coronal suture is demonstrated, frontal bossing and the low nasal bridge are clearly demonstrated

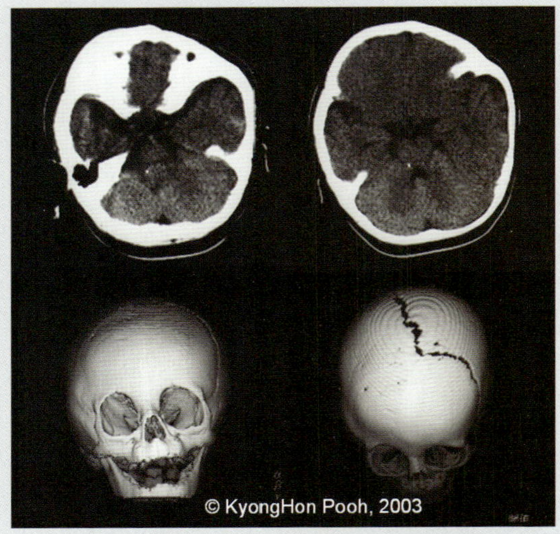

Figure 6.74 Plagiocephaly with synostosis of unilateral coronal suture. Upper, CT scan images. Skull deformity is seen. Lower, three-dimensional reconstruction CT images. Complete fusion of right coronal suture is demonstrated

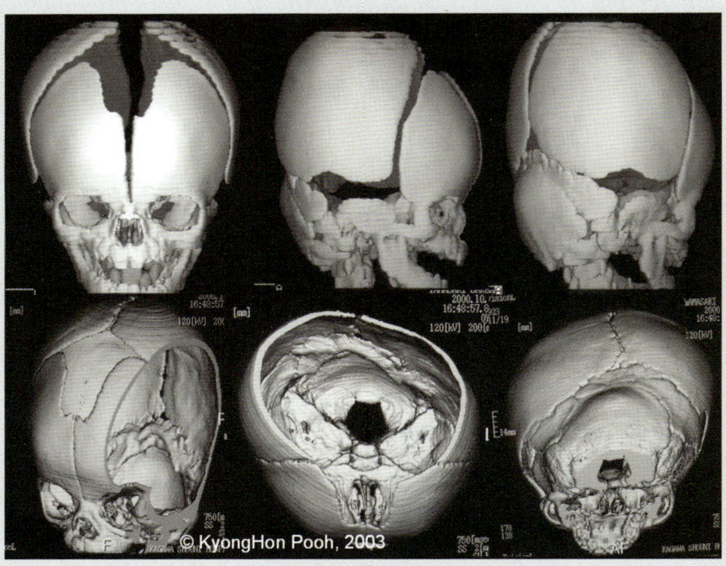

Figure 6.73 Three-dimensional reconstruction CT images of acrocephaly with synostosis of lamboid sutures (same case as shown in Figure 6.72). Upper, external views of the cranium. Note the fusion of the lamboid sutures. Lower, internal views of the cranium

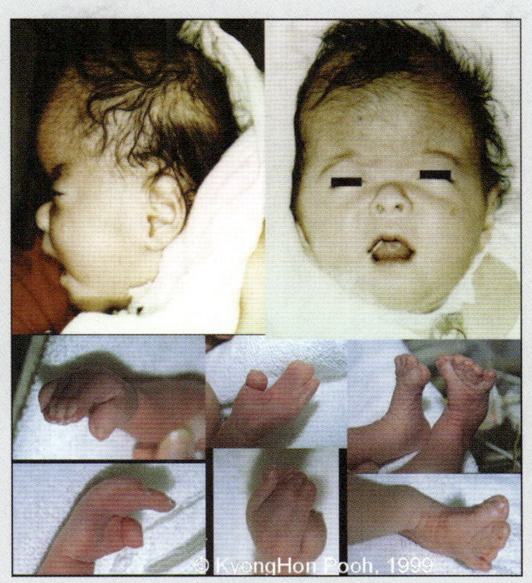

Figure 6.75 Apert syndrome (same case as shown in Figure 6.71 of prenatal images). Upper, appearance of brachycephaly due to bilateral fused coronal sutures. Tracheostomy was performed for respiratory tract stenosis due to severe deformed craniofacial bony dysplasia. Lower, syndactyly of hands and feet bilaterally, which is characteristic of Apert syndrome

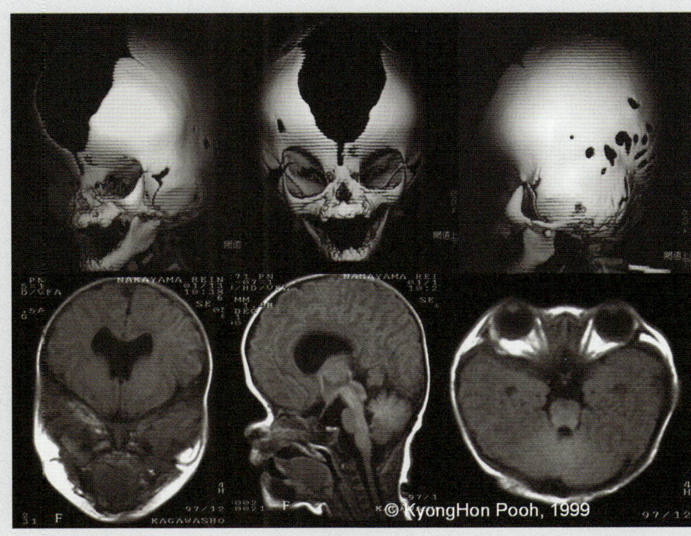

Figure 6.76 Three-dimensional reconstruction CT and magnetic resonance images of Apert syndrome (same case as shown in Figures 6.71 and 6.75). Upper, three-dimensional reconstruction CT. Fusion of bilateral coronal suture and squamous suture, defect of frontoparietal cranial structure and craniofacial bony dysplasia are recognizable. Lower, magnetic resonance images. Marked shortening of anterior cranial fossa is seen. Mild ventriculomegaly and absent septum pellucidum are present

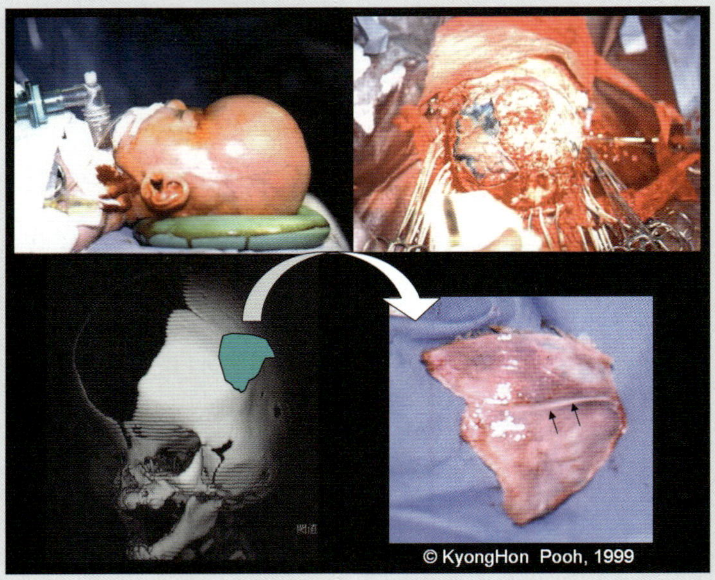

Figure 6.77 Cranioplasty of Apert syndrome (same case as shown in Figures 6.71, 6.75 and 6.76). Upper left, conspicuous frontal bossing and low nasal bridge. Upper right, photograph during cranioplasty. Lower left, three-dimensional CT before operation showing position of bone seen in right photograph. Lower right, inside view of the resected part of cranial bone including synostosis of the coronal suture. Arrows indicate the fused coronal suture

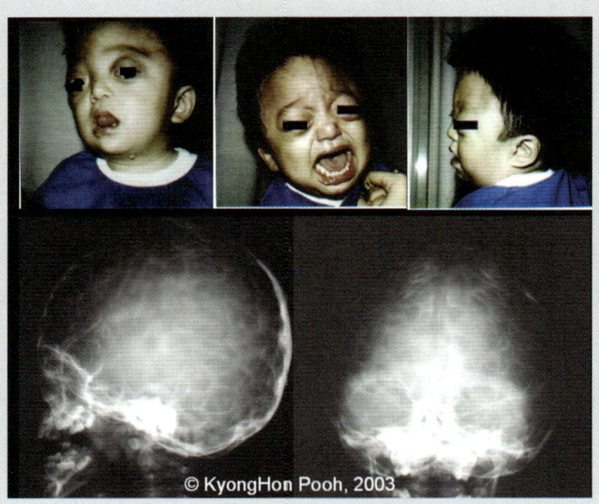

Figure 6.78 Crouzon disease. Upper, facial appearance. Exophthalmos and deformed craniofacial shape are seen. Lower, roentgenogram. Oxycephaly is demonstrated by total sutural fusion

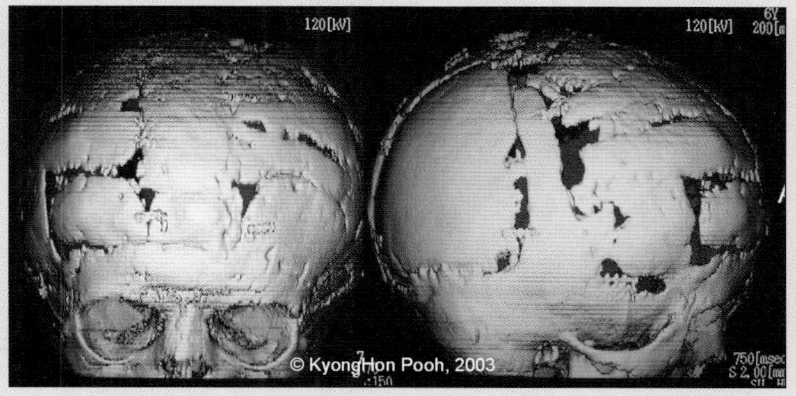

Figure 6.79 Postnatal three-dimensional reconstruction CT in case of Crouzon disease (same case as shown in Figure 6.78). Radical reconstructive cranioplasty was performed

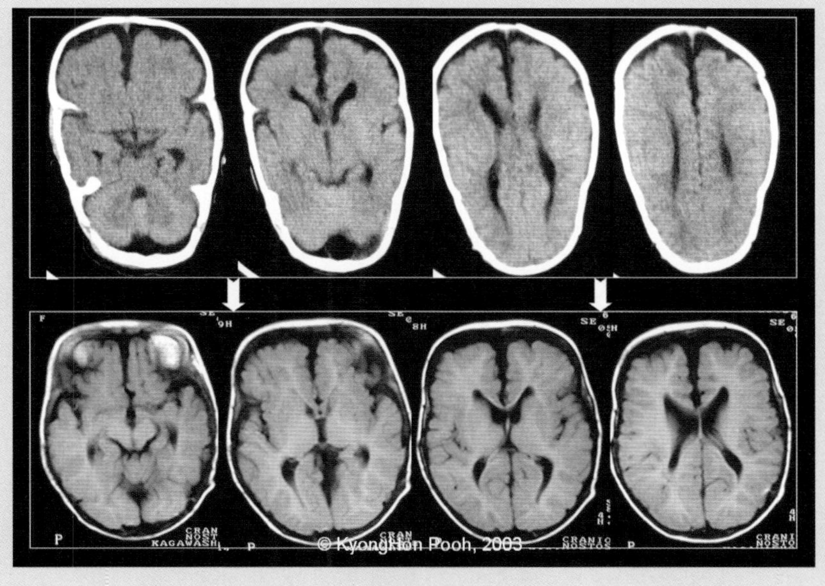

Figure 6.80 Treatment of scaphocephaly (synostosis of sagittal suture). Upper, preoperative CT axial images. Skull development toward temporal direction is prevented, especially in the occipital portion. Lower, postoperative magnetic resonance axial images. After cranioplasty, scaphocephalic shape and cerebral compression improved

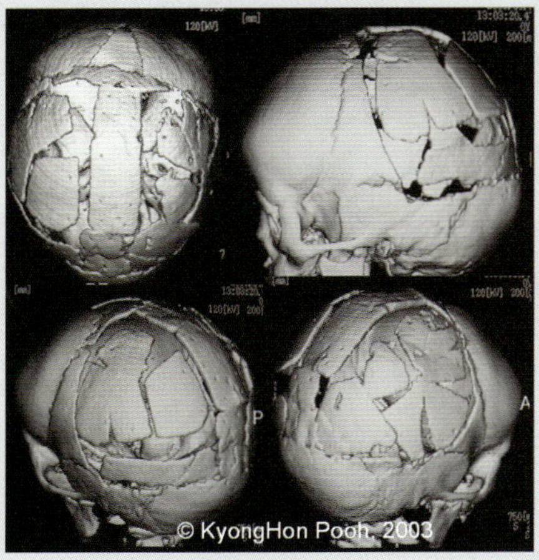

Figure 6.81 Three-dimensional reconstruction CT images after cranioplasty in a case of scaphocephaly (same case as shown in Figure 6.80)

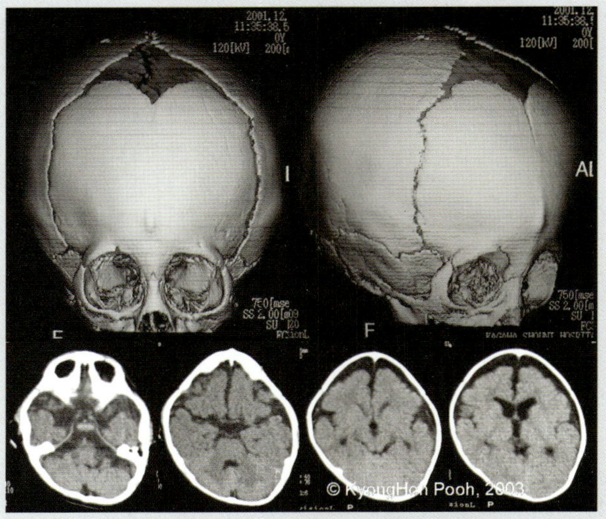

Figure 6.82 Trigonocephaly with synostosis of metopic suture. Upper, preoperative three-dimensional reconstruction CT images. Metopic suture is completely fused. Lower, CT scan images of trigonocephaly. Note the triangular shape of the forehead

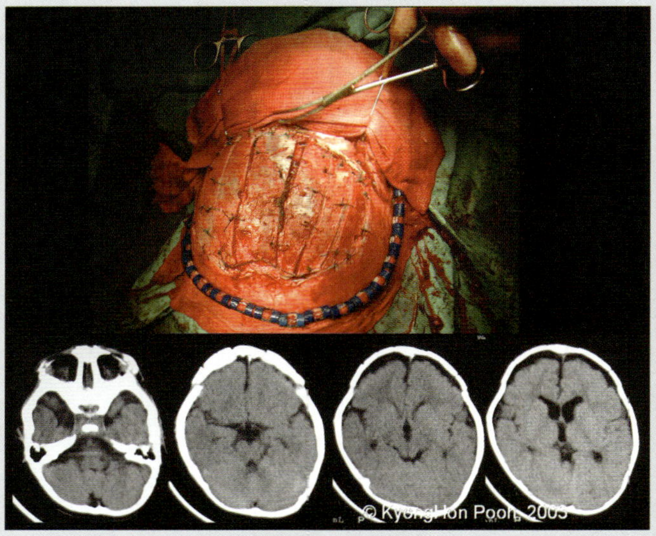

Figure 6.83 Treatment of trigonocephaly (same case as shown in Figure 6.82). Upper, photograph during cranioplastic operation. Lower, postoperative CT images. Skull deformity improved by cranioplasty

(3) *Pfeiffer syndrome* Brachycephaly, synostosis of coronal and/or sagittal sutures; with hypertelorism, broad thumbs and toes, partial syndactyly.

(4) *Antley–Bixler syndrome* Brachycephaly, multiple synostosis, especially of coronal suture; with maxillary hypoplasia, radiohymeral synostosis, choanal atresia, arthrogryposis.

Etiology Crouzon (autosomal dominant, variable), Apert (autosomal dominant, usually new mutation), Pfeiffer (autosomal dominant), Antley–Bixler (autosomal recessive). Five autosomal dominant craniosynostosis syndromes (Apert, Crouzon, Pfeiffer, Jackson–Weiss and Crouzon syndrome with acanthosis nigricans) result from mutations in *FGFR* genes[35].

Pathogenesis

(1) Cranial vault bones with decreased growth potential;

(2) Asymmetrical bone deposition at perimeter sutures;

(3) Sutures adjacent to the prematurely fused suture compensate in growth more than those sutures not contiguous with the closed suture;

(4) Enhanced symmetrical bone deposition occurs along both sides of a non-perimeter suture continuing a prematurely closed suture.

Associated anomalies Hypertelorism, syndactyly, polydactyly, exophthalmos.

Prenatal diagnosis Figures 6.71 and 6.72. Abnormal craniofacial appearance by two- and three-dimensional ultrasound[37,38].

Prognosis Various. In some trigonocephaly and syndromic types, prognosis is poor.

Recurrence risk Depends on etiology.

Management The operative aim of cranioplasty is the improvement of intracranial pressure and cosmetic change (Figures 6.75–6.83).

OTHERS

Vein of Galen aneurysm (Figures 6.84 and 6.85)

Incidence Rare.

Definition Direct arteriovenous fistulas between choroidal and/or quadrigeminal arteries and an overlying single median venous sac.

Synonyms Vein of Galen malformation.

Etiology Unknown.

Pathogenesis Venous sac most probably represents persistence of the embryonic median prosencephalic vein of Markowski, not the vein of Galen, *per se*[39].

Associated anomalies Cardiomegaly, high cardiac output, secondary hydrocephalus, macrocrania, cerebral ischemia (intracranial steal phenomenon), subarachnoid/cerebral/intraventricular hemorrhages.

Prenatal diagnosis Figures 6.84 and 6.85.

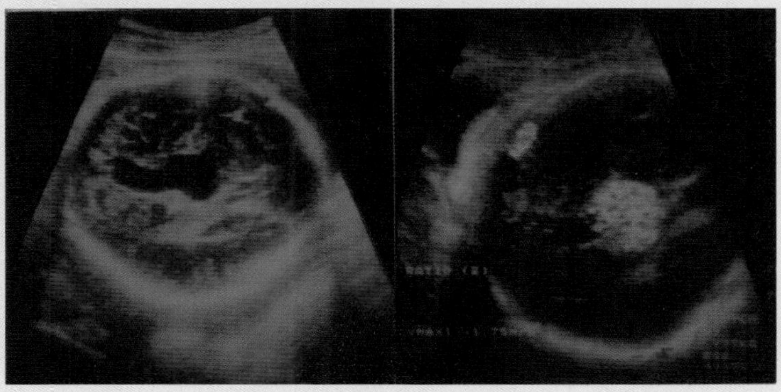

Figure 6.84 Vein of Galen aneurysm at 35 weeks of gestation. Left, large Galen aneurysm and straight sinus are demonstrated. Right, mosaic flow inside the aneurysm is demonstrated by a Color Doppler image. Image courtesy of Dr M. Utsu

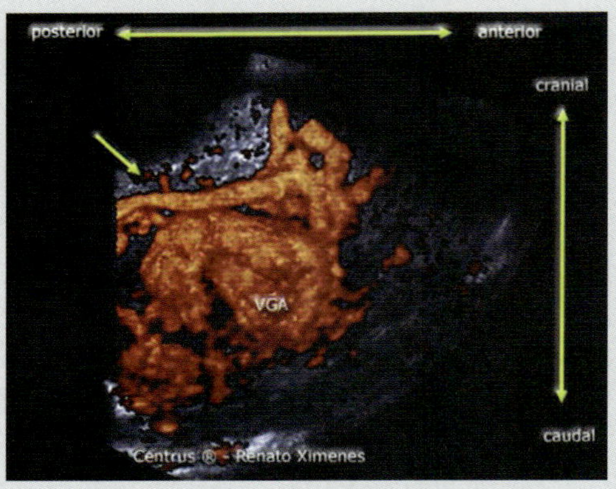

Figure 6.85 Galen aneurysm at 35 weeks of gestation. This is the third-trimester fetus with a large vein of Galen aneurysm (VGA). The three-dimensional power angio reconstruction demonstrates well the chaotic appearance and connections of the feeder and draining vessels. Image courtesy of Dr X. Renato, www.TheFetus.net, with permission

Differential diagnosis Arachnoid cyst, porencephalic cyst, intracranial teratoma. Color/power Doppler is helpful for differential diagnosis.

Prognosis According to an earlier review, outcome did not differ between treated and non-treated groups and over 80% of the cases died[40]. However, recent advances in treatment have improved outcome, such that 60–100% survive and over 60% have a good neurological outcome[41,42].

Recurrence risk Unknown.

Management Evaluation of the fetal high-output cardiac state for proper obstetric management. Percutaneous embolization by microcoils is the recent main postnatal treatment with remarkably improved outcome.

Arachnoid cyst (Figures 6.86–6.101)

Prevalence 1% of intracranial masses in newborns.

Definition Congenital or acquired cyst, lined by arachnoid membranes, and filled with fluid collection which is the same character as CSF. The number of cysts is mostly single, but two or more cysts can occasionally be observed. Location of an arachnoid

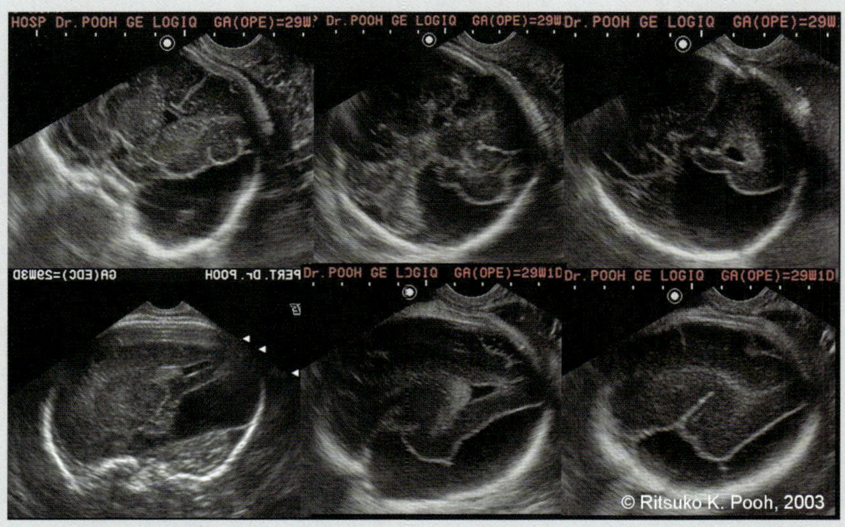

Figure 6.86 Transvaginal ultrasound images of an arachnoid cyst at 29 weeks of gestation. Upper, serial coronal sections. Lower, serial sagittal sections. A compressed adjacent cerebrum is demonstrated

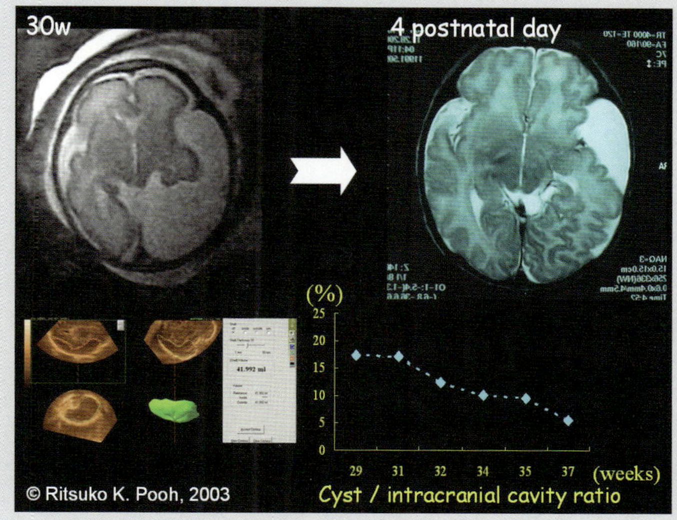

Figure 6.87 Intrauterine spontaneous resolution of an arachnoid cyst (same case as shown in Figure 6.86). Spontaneous size reduction was observed during pregnancy. Upper left, fetal magnetic resonance image (MRI) at 30 weeks. Upper right, neonatal MRI at 4th postnatal day. Lower left, three-dimensional ultrasound volume calculation of the arachnoid cyst. Lower right, cyst/intracranial cavity ratio between 29 and 37 weeks of gestation

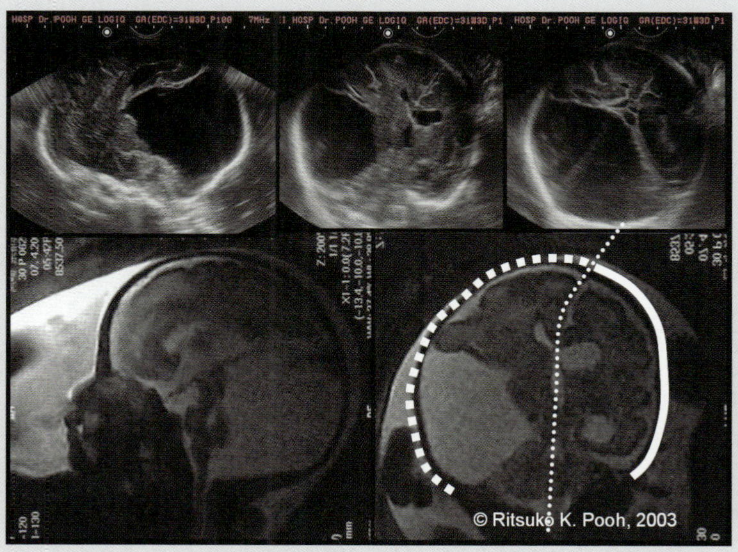

Figure 6.88 Fetal arachnoid cyst at 31 weeks of gestation. Upper, transvaginal ultrasound image; sagittal (left) and coronal (middle, right) sections. Lower left, fetal magnetic resonance sagittal image. The cyst occupies supra- to infratentorial space. Not only the cerebrum but also the cerebellum are compressed by the cyst. Lower right, fetal magnetic resonance coronal image. Midline is conspicuously arcuated. Scalp and skull bone are extended due to the existence of the huge cyst. Note the difference between the right and left head size

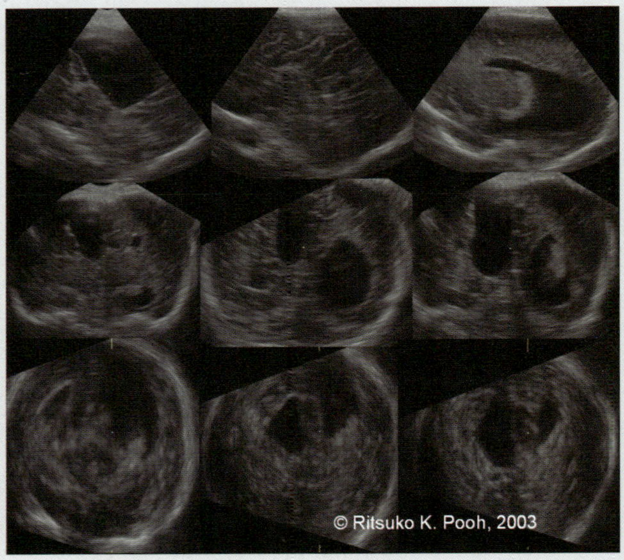

Figure 6.89 Fetal ultrasound images of an interhemispheric cyst associated with agenesis of the corpus callosum. Upper, serial sagittal images. Radiated sulci formation and colpocephaly are demonstrated. Middle, serial coronal images. Unilateral ventriculomegaly is clearly seen. Lower, serial axial images

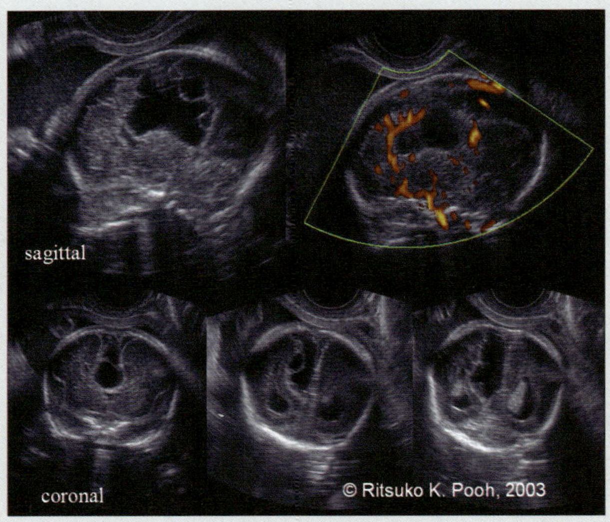

Figure 6.90 Fetal ultrasound images of an interhemispheric cyst with hypogenesis of the corpus callosum at 24 weeks of gestation. All images are by the transvaginal approach. Upper left, sagittal section. The cyst is not a simple cyst but contains a thin septal membrane and several small cysts inside. Upper right, power Doppler imaging in the sagittal section. It is hard to observe the corpus callosum in a B-mode sonogram; however, the fact that a pericallosal artery is depicted may indicate hypogenesis of the corpus callosum not agenesis. Lower, serial transvaginal coronal images

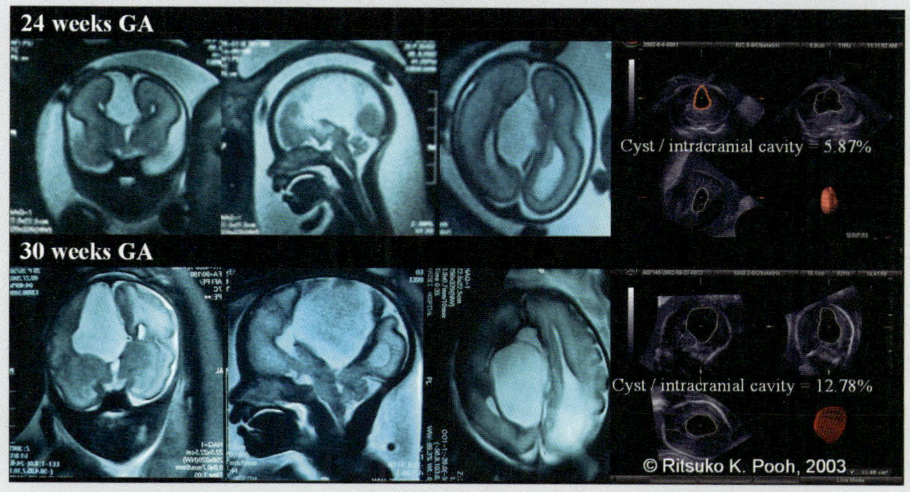

Figure 6.91 Fetal magnetic resonance images and three-dimensional ultrasound volume calculation of an interhemispheric cyst with hypogenesis of the corpus callosum at 24 and 30 weeks of gestation (same case as shown in Figure 6.90). Upper, 24 weeks of gestation. The cyst occupying ratio is 5.87%. Lower, 30 weeks of gestation. The cyst occupying ratio is 12.78%; gradual progression of the cyst is demonstrated. In this case, spontaneous reduction in size of the cyst was seen after birth. GA, gestational age

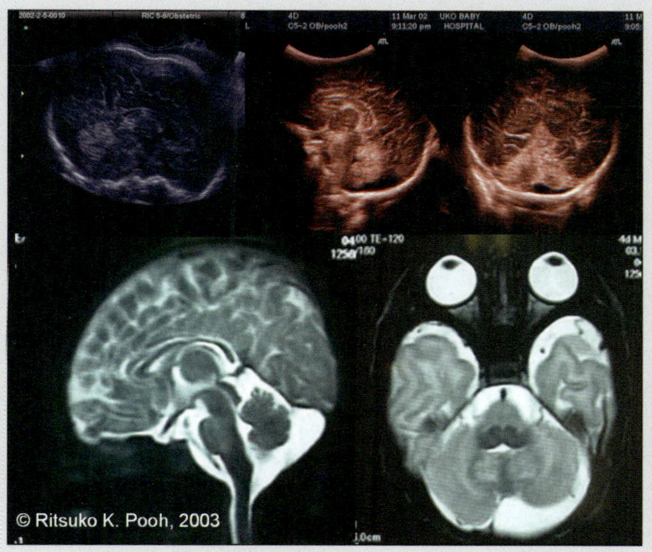

Figure 6.92 An arachnoid cyst in the posterior fossa. Upper left, fetal ultrasound sagittal image. A megacisterna magna was the prenatal diagnosis. Upper middle and right, neonatal ultrasound sagittal and coronal images. Note the asymmetrical cisterna magna. Lower, neonatal magnetic resonance sagittal and axial images. The cystic formation in the cisterna magna affects the asymmetry of the cerebellar hemispheres

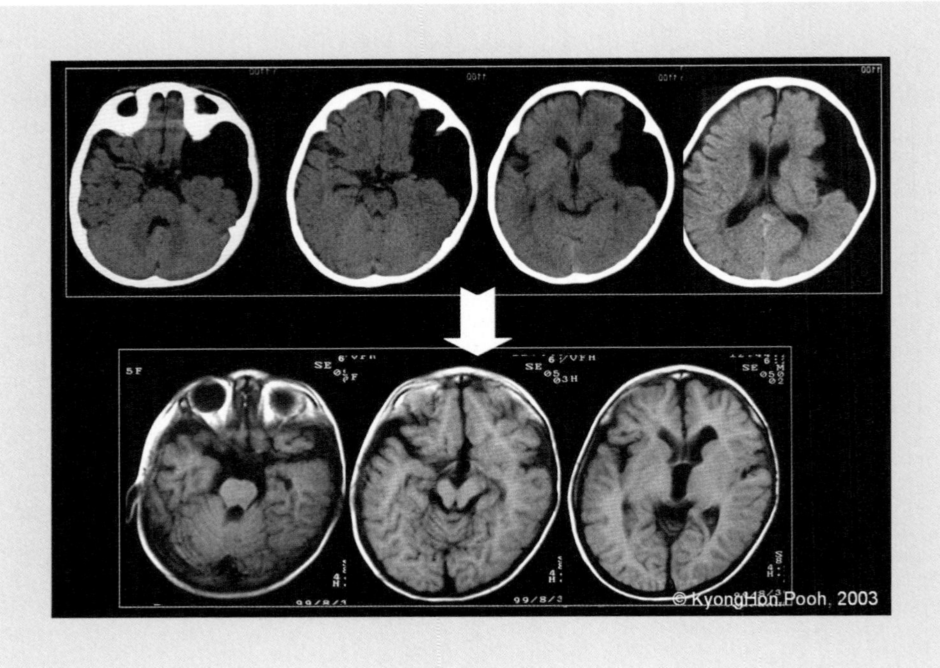

Figure 6.93 Fenestration under craniotomy of a neonatal arachnoid cyst. Upper, magnetic resonance axial images of a sylvian fissure (middle fossa) arachnoid cyst, before operation. Lower, postoperative magnetic resonance image. Fenestration by craniotomy was selected in this case. Communication to the basal cistern by cyst fenestration resulted in regression of the cyst. The postoperative course has been uneventful for 1 year

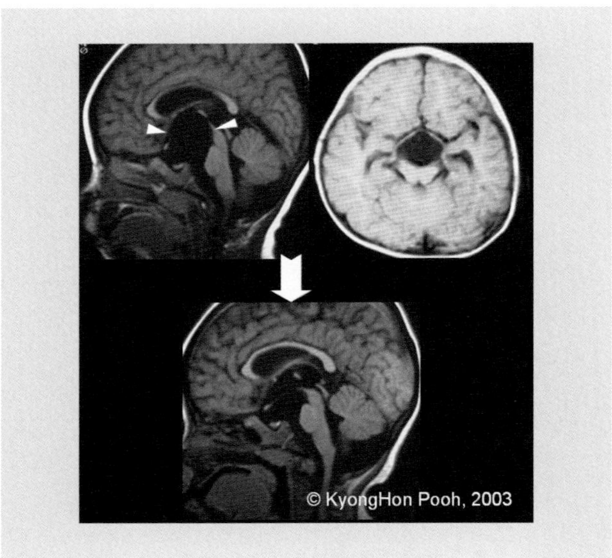

Figure 6.94 Fenestration by neuroendoscopy of a suprasellar arachnoid cyst. Upper left, before operation, a magnetic resonance sagittal image shows that the suprasellar arachnoid cyst (arrowhead) compresses the mid-brain. Upper right, although hydrocephalus is often a complication, no ventriculomegaly is seen in this case. Lower, postoperative magnetic resonance sagittal image. After fenestration by neuroendoscopy, the cyst size was reduced

cyst is various; approximately 50% of cysts occur from the Sylvian fissure (middle fossa), 20% from the posterior fossa and 10–20% each from the convexity, suprasellar, interhemisphere and quadrigeminal cistern. Interhemispheric cysts are often associated with agenesis or hypogenesis of the corpus callosum.

Etiology Unknown.

Pathogenesis A congenital arachnoid cyst is formed by maldevelopment of the arachnoid membrane. CSF accumulation in the subarachnoid space or intra-arachnoid layers from a choroid plexus-like tissue within the cyst wall, leads to a progressive distention of the lesion.

Associated anomalies Unilateral or bilateral hydrocephalus, macrocrania.

Prenatal diagnosis Figures 6.86–6.92. Detection in the first trimester has been reported[43].

Differential diagnosis Porencephaly, schizencephaly, third ventriculomegaly, intracranial cystic type tumor, vein of Galen aneurysm, Dandy–Walker malformation, large cisterna magna and external hydrocephalus.

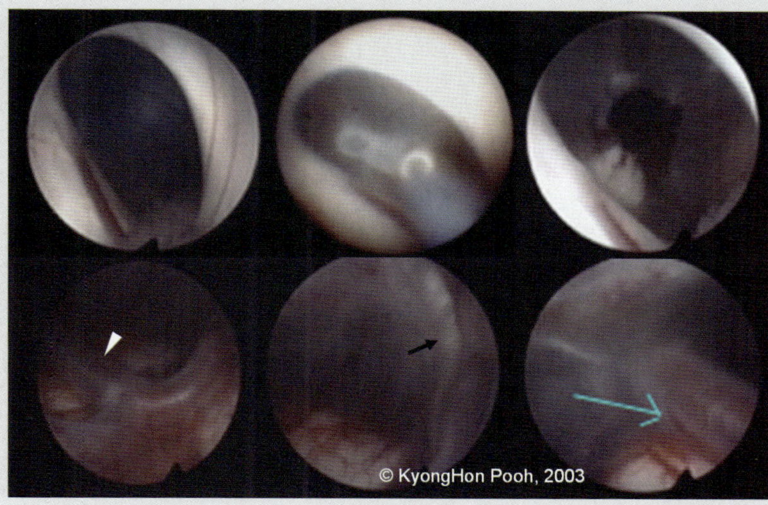

Figure 6.95 Neuroendoscopic views (same case as shown in Figure 6.94). Upper left, most of the foramen of Monro was obstructed by the arachnoid cyst wall. Upper middle, coagulating the cyst wall by monopolar coagulator. Upper right, after fenestration of the cyst wall. Lower left, inside the cyst; observation of the basal cistern through the floor of the arachnoid cyst. The basilar artery (arrowhead) is seen. Lower middle, the left side of the lower left image. The oculomotor nerve (black arrow) is observed. Lower right, the blue arrow indicates slit-like tear of the cyst wall, adjacent to the basilar artery. The existence of this slit, as a one-way valve, may have led to cyst expansion before treatment

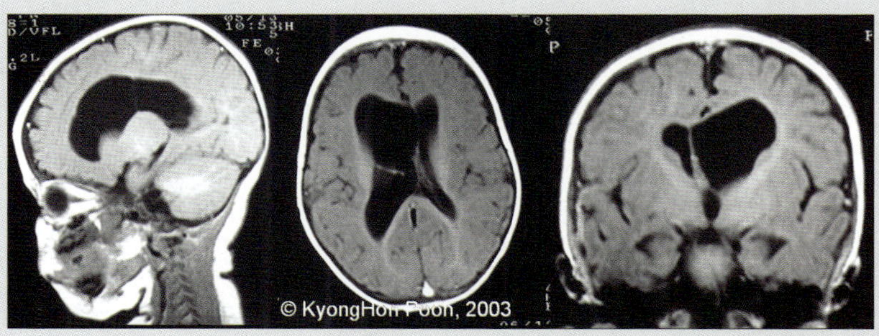

Figure 6.96 Intraventricular cyst (postnatal magnetic resonance image). Magnetic resonance sagittal, axial and coronal images from left side. The thin cyst wall is demonstrated inside the unilateral ventricle. Obstruction of the foramen of Monro by the cyst wall may cause unilateral ventriculomegaly

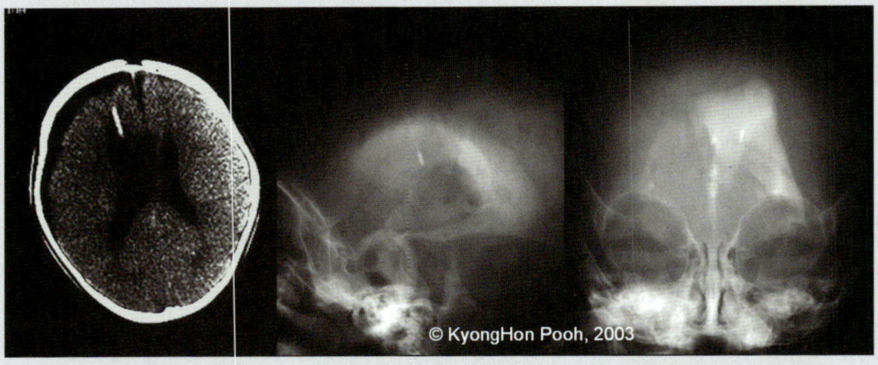

Figure 6.97 Fenestration of an intraventricular cyst by neuroendoscopy (same case as shown in Figure 6.96). Left, postoperative CT image. Cyst fenestration under neuroendoscopy results in regression of ventriculomegaly. Middle, right, postoperative ventriculogram. Communication between the cyst and lateral ventricle is demonstrated

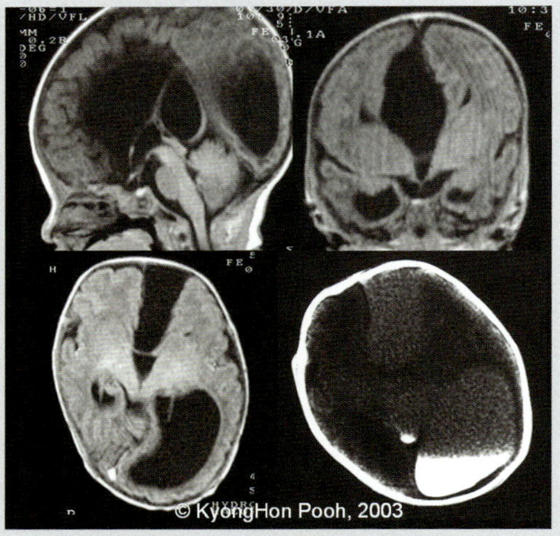

Figure 6.98 Interhemispheric cyst complicated with agenesis of the corpus callosum (neonatal magnetic resonance image). Obstruction of the foramen of Monro unilaterally by an interhemispheric cyst causes unilateral hydrocephalus. Upper left, magnetic resonance sagittal image. Upper right, magnetic resonance coronal image. Note the bull horn shape of the anterior horns of the lateral ventricles, which is one of the characteristics of agenesis of the corpus callosum. Lower left, magnetic resonance axial image. Unilateral hydrocephalus is demonstrated. Lower right, CT ventriculography indicates existence of communication between the right ventricle and the interhemispheric cyst

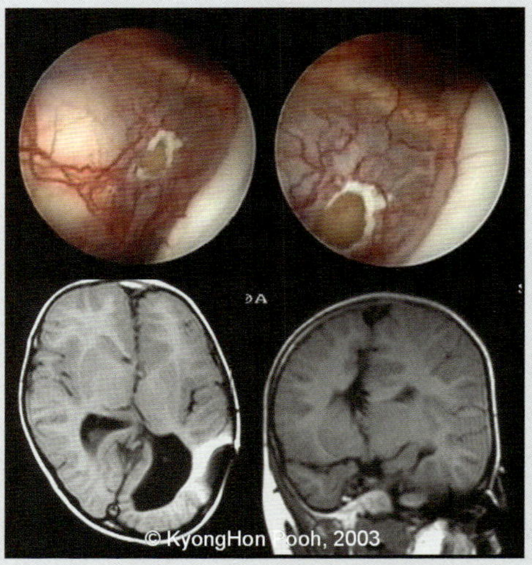

Figure 6.99 Treatment of an interhemispheric cyst (same case as shown in Figure 6.98). Upper, neuroendoscopic view. The cyst was communicated to the third ventricle by fenestration. The fenestration window is visible. In this case, a ventriculoperitoneal shunt was added because the fenestration window was occluded. Lower, magnetic resonance axial and coronal images after treatment. Regression of the interhemispheric cyst and unilateral hydrocephalus is demonstrated

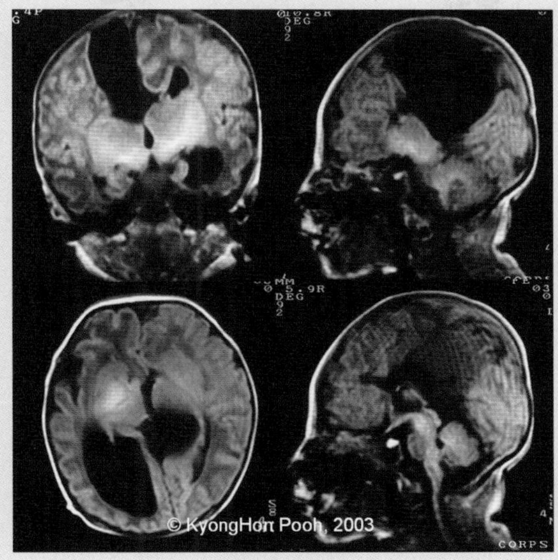

Figure 6.100 Postnatal magnetic resonance images of an interhemispheric cyst associated with agenesis of the corpus callosum (same case as shown in Figure 6.89). Upper left, coronal image. Upper right, sagittal image. An interhemispheric cyst is clearly demonstrated. Lower left, axial image. Unilateral ventriculomegaly is demonstrated. Lower right, median image. The corpus callosum is absent

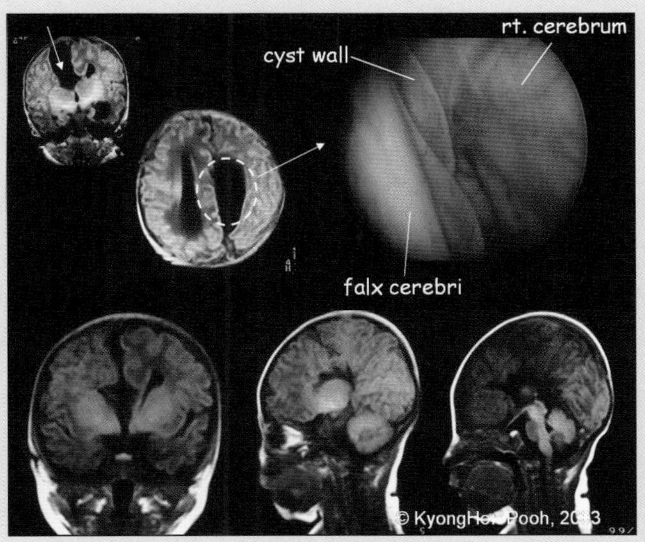

Figure 6.101 Neuroendoscopy for a neonatal interhemispheric cyst (same case as shown in Figures 6.89 and 6.100). Upper left, neonatal magnetic resonance images. The neuroendoscopic procedure is done through the parietal roof of the interhemispheric cyst. Right, neuroendoscopic view. The thin membranous cyst wall, falx cerebri and surface of the right cerebrum are visible. Total cyst resection was performed by using endoscopy. Lower, postoperative magnetic resonance image. The interhemispheric cyst was completely resected and the typical appearance of agenesis of the corpus callosum is demonstrated

Prognosis Generally good. Postnatally, many are asymptomatic and remain quiescent for years, although others expand and cause neurological symptoms by compressing the adjacent brain, ventriculomegaly and/or expanding the overlying skull.

Recurrence risk Unknown.

Obstetric management Arachnoid cysts may increase or decrease their size (Figures 6.87–6.91). Therefore, expectant management of antenatally diagnosed cases is suggested[44]. In cases with accompanying hydrocephalus, mode and timing of delivery may be modified.

Postnatal management Figures 6.93–6.101. In cases with these symptoms or with prospects of neurological symptoms, treatment should be considered. Operation methods include cyst fenestration by craniotomy, cyst fenestration by neuroendoscopy and cyst–peritoneal shunt. Craniotomy, shunting or the neuroendoscopic method are still controversial[45,46].

Choroid plexus cysts (Figures 6.102 and 6.103)

Incidence 0.95–2.8% of all fetuses scanned[47–49].

Definition Cysts with fluid collection within the choroid plexus, which may exist unilaterally or bilaterally. They are depicted in the second trimester and usually resolve by the 24th week.

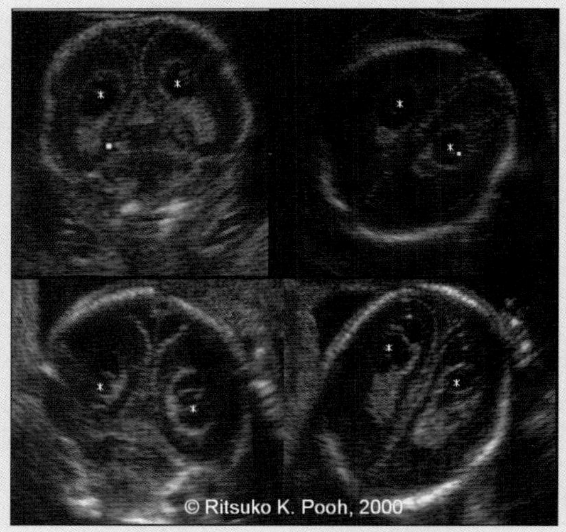

Figure 6.102 Fetal ultrasound images of choroid plexus cysts. Upper, bilateral choroid plexus cysts in a fetus with trisomy 18. Cardiac ventricular septum defect and overlapping fingers were present. Lower, bilateral choroid plexus cysts in a normal fetus. It is impossible to differentiate between normal and abnormal karyotypes by location and appearance of a choroid plexus cyst. Detection of additional anomalies is important for a differential diagnosis

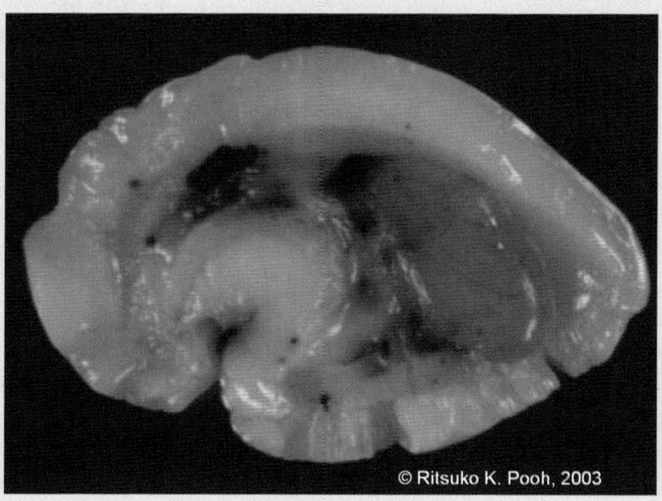

Figure 6.103 Macroscopic appearance of a choroid plexus cyst in an aborted fetus with trisomy 18 at 20 weeks of gestation

Etiology Normal variant, chromosomal aberration such as trisomy 18 and others.

Pathogenesis The choroid plexus is located within the ventricular system and produces cerebrospinal fluid. Within the choroidal villi, choroid plexus cysts exist, surrounded by the loose stroma of the choroid plexus[50].

Associated anomalies In cases of trisomy 18, associated anomalies include growth restriction, congenital heart diseases such as ventricular septum defect and double outlet right ventricle, overlapping finger, facial anomaly, cerebellar dysplasia and others.

Prenatal diagnosis Figure 6.102; macroscopic appearence is shown in Figure 6.103.

Differential diagnosis Intraventricular hemorrhage.

Prognosis Choroid plexus cysts, per se, are usually asymptomatic and benign, but rarely, are symptomatic and disturb CSF flow[51,52]. Isolated choroid plexus cysts may be a normal variation.

Recurrence risk Unknown.

Management Fetal karyotyping examination should be offered if additional abnormalities are found.

REFERENCES

1. Martinez de Villarreal L, Perez JZ, *et al.* Decline of neural tube defects cases after a folic acid campaign in Nuevo Leon, Mexico. *Teratology* 2002;66:249–56
2. Ray JG, Meier C, Vermeulen MJ, *et al.* Association of neural tube defects and folic acid food fortification in Canada. *Lancet* 2002;360:2047–8
3. Green NS. Folic acid supplementation and prevention of birth defects. *J Nutr* 2002;132:2356S–60S
4. Persad VL, Van den Hof MC, Dube JM, *et al.* Incidence of open neural tube defects in Nova Scotia after folic acid fortification. *CMAJ* 2002;167:241–5
5. Mathews TJ, Honein MA, Erickson JD. Spina bifida and anencephaly prevalence – United States, 1991–2001. *MMWR Recomm Rep* 2002;51:9–11
6. Stevenson RE, Allen WP, Pai GS, *et al.* Decline in prevalence of neural tube defects in a high-risk region of the United States. *Pediatrics* 2000;106:677–83
7. Monteagudo A, Timor-Tritsch IE. Fetal neurosonography of congenital brain anomalies. In Timor-Tritsch IE, Monteagudo A, Cohen HL, eds. *Ultrasonography of the Prenatal and Neonatal Brain.* 2nd edn. New York: McGraw-Hill, 2001:151–258
8. Matsunaga E, Shiota K. Holoprosencephaly in hyman embryos: epidemiologic studies of 150 cases. *Teratology* 1977;16:261–72
9. Cohen MM Jr. Perspectives on holoprosencephaly. I. Epidemiology, genetics and syndromology. *Teratology* 1989;40:211–35
10. Volpe JJ. Neural tube formation and prosencephalic development. In *Neurology of the Newborn*. 4th edn. Philadelphia: W.B. Saunders, 2001:3–44
11. Pilu G, Ambrosetto P, Sandri F, *et al.* Intraventricular fused fornices: a specific sign of fetal lobar holoprosencephaly. *Ultrasound Obstet Gynecol* 1994;34: 259–62
12. Cohen MM. An update on the holoprosencephalic disorders. *J Pediatr* 1982;101:865–9
13. Pilu G, Porelo A, Falco P, *et al.* Median anomalies of the brain. In Timor-Tritsch IE, Monteagudo A, Cohen HL, eds. *Ultrasonography of the Prenatal and Neonatal Brain.* 2nd edn. New York: McGraw-Hill, 2001:259–76
14. Goodyear PW, Bannister CM, Russell S, *et al.* Outcome in prenatally diagnosed fetal agenesis of the corpus callosum. *Fetal Diagn Ther* 2001;16:139–45
15. Taylor M, David AS. Agenesis of the corpus callosum: a United Kingdom series of 56 cases. *J Neurol Neurosurg Psychiatr* 1998;64:131–4
16. Schmidt-Riese U, Zieger M. Ultrasound diagnosis of isolated aplasia of the septum pellucidum. *Ultraschall Med* 1994;15:286–92
17. McMahon CL, Braddock SR. Septo-optic dysplasia as a manifestation of valproic acid embryopathy. *Teratology* 2001;64:83–6
18. Dominguez R, Aguirre Vila-Coro A, Slopis JM, *et al.* Brain and ocular abnormalities in infants with *in utero* exposure to cocaine and other street drugs. *Am J Dis Child* 1991;145:688–95
19. Dattani MT, Martinez-Barbera JP, Thomas PQ, *et al.* Mutations in the homeobox gene *HESX1/Hesx1* associated with septo-optic dysplasia in human and mouse. *Nat Genet* 1998;19:125–33
20. Volpe JJ. Neuronal proliferation, migration, organization and myelination. In *Neurology of the Newborn.* 4th edn. Philadelphia: W.B. Saunders, 2001:45–99
21. Kobayashi K, Nakahori Y, Miyake M, *et al.* An ancient retrotransposal insertion causes Fukuyama-type congenital muscular dystrophy. *Nature* 1998;394:388–92
22. McGahan JP, Grix A, Gerscovich EO. Prenatal diagnosis of lissencephaly: Miller–Dieker syndrome. *J Clin Ultrasound* 1994;22:560–3
23. Greco P, Resta M, Vimercati A, *et al.* Antenatal diagnosis of isolated lissencephaly by ultrasound and

magnetic resonance imaging. *Ultrasound Obstet Gynecol* 1998;12:276–9

24. Kojima K, Suzuki Y, Seki K, *et al.* Prenatal diagnosis of lissencephaly (type II) by ultrasound and fast magnetic resonance imaging. *Fetal Diagn Ther* 2002;17:34–6

25. Granata T, Farina L, Faiella A, *et al.* Familial schizencephaly associated with *EMX2* mutation. *Neurology* 1997;48:1403–6

26. Brunelli S, Faiella A, Capra V, *et al.* Germline mutations in the homeobox gene *EMX2* in patients with severe schizencephaly. *Nat Genet* 1996;12:94–6

27. Iannetti P, Nigro G, Spalice A, *et al.* Cytomegalovirus infection and schizencephaly: case reports. *Ann Neurol* 1998;43:123–7

28. Denis D, Maugey-Laulom B, Carles D, *et al.* Prenatal diagnosis of schizencephaly by fetal magnetic resonance imaging. *Fetal Diagn Ther* 2001;16:354–9

29. Osenbach RK, Menezes AH. Diagnosis and management of the Dandy–Walker malformation: 30 years of experience. *Pediatr Neurosurg* 1991;18:179–85

30. Barkovich AJ, Kjos BO, Normal D, *et al.* Revised classification of the posterior fossa cysts and cyst-like malformations based on the results of multiplanar MR imaging. *AJNR* 1989;10:977–88

31. D'Addario V, Pinto V, Del Bianco A, *et al.* The clivus-supraocciput angle: a useful measurement to evaluate the shape and size of the fetal posterior fossa and to diagnose Chiari II malformation. *Ultrasound Obstet Gynecol* 2001;18:146–9

32. Utsunomiya H, Takano K, Ogasawara T, *et al.* Rhombencephalosynapsis: cerebellar embryogenesis. *AJNR Am J Neuroradiol* 1998;19:547–9

33. Yachnis AT. Rhombencephalosynapsis with massive hydrocephalus: case report and pathogenetic considerations. *Acta Neuropathol* 2002;103:301–4

34. Toelle SP, Yalcinkaya C, Kocer N, *et al.* Rhombencephalosynapsis: clinical findings and neuroimaging in 9 children. *Neuropediatrics* 2002;33:209–14

35. Hollway GE, Suthers GK, Haan EA, *et al.* Mutation detection in *FGFR2* craniosynostosis syndromes. *Hum Genet* 1997;99:251–5

36. Delashaw JB, Persing JA, Broaddus WC, *et al.* Cranial vault growth in craniosynostosis. *J Neurosurg* 1989;70:159–65

37. Benacerraf BR, Spiro R, Mitchell AG. Using three-dimensional ultrasound to detect craniosynostosis in a fetus with Pfeiffer syndrome. *Ultrasound Obstet Gynecol* 2000;16:391–4

38. Pooh RK, Nakagawa Y, Pooh KH, *et al.* Fetal craniofacial structure and intracranial morphology in a case of Apert syndrome. *Ultrasound Obstet Gynecol* 1999;13:274–80

39. Raybaud CA, Strother CM, Hald JK. Aneurysms of the vein of Galen: embryonic considerations and anatomical features relating to the pathogenesis of the malformation. *Neuroradiology* 1989;31:109–28

40. Hoffman HJ, Chuang S, Hendrick EB, *et al.* Aneurysms of the vein of Galen. Experience at The Hospital for Sick Children, Toronto. *J Neurosurg* 1982;57:316–22

41. Campi A, Rodesch G, Scotti G, *et al.* Aneurysmal malformation of the vein of Galen in three patients: clinical and radiological follow-up. *Neuroradiology* 1998;40:816–21

42. Friedman DM, Verma R, Madrid M, *et al.* Recent improvement in outcome using transcatheter embolization techniques for neonatal aneurysmal malformations of the vein of Galen. *Pediatrics* 1993;91:583–6

43. Bretelle F, Senat MV, Bernard JP, *et al.* First-trimester diagnosis of fetal arachnoid cyst: prenatal implication. *Ultrasound Obstet Gynecol* 2002;20:400–2

44. Elbers SE, Furness ME. Resolution of presumed arachnoid cyst *in utero*. *Ultrasound Obstet Gynecol* 1999;14:353–5

45. Ciricillo SF, Cogen PH, Harsh GR, *et al.* Intracranial arachnoid cysts in children. A comparison of the effects of fenestration and shunting. *J Neurosurg* 1991;74:230–5

46. Nakamura Y, Mizukawa K, Yamamoto K, *et al.* Endoscopic treatment for a huge neonatal prepontine–suprasellar arachnoid cyst: a case report. *Pediatr Neurosurg* 2001;35:220–4

47. Sullivan A, Giudice T, Vavelidis F, *et al.* Choroid plexus cysts: is biochemical testing a valuable adjunct to targeted ultrasonography? *Am J Obstet Gynecol* 1999;181:260–5

48. Reinsch RC. Choroid plexus cysts – association with trisomy: prospective review of 16 059 patients. *Am J Obstet Gynecol* 1997;176:1381–3

49. Morcos CL, Platt LD, Carlson DE, *et al.* The isolated choroid plexus cyst. *Obstet Gynecol* 1998;92:232–6

50. Farhood AI, Morris JH, Bieber FR. Transient cysts of the fetal choroid plexus: morphology and histogenesis. *Am J Med Genet* 1987;27:977–82

51. Lam AH, Villanueva AC. Symptomatic third ventricular choroid plexus cysts. *Pediatr Radiol* 1992;22:413–16

52. Parizek J, Jakubec J, Hobza V, *et al.* Choroid plexus cyst of the left lateral ventricle with intermittent blockage of the foramen of Monro, and initial invagination into the III ventricle in a child. *Childs Nerv Syst* 1998;14:700–8

7

Acquired brain abnormalities *in utero*

R.K. Pooh, K. Maeda and K.H. Pooh

SUBEPENDYMAL PSEUDOCYSTS

Prevalence 2.6–5% of all neonates, 1% of premature newborns, unknown in fetuses.

Definition Cystic formation, which is located in the caudothalamic groove or in the caudate nucleus, lateral to the wall of the anterior horns of lateral ventricles.

Synonyms Periventricular pseudocysts[1,2].

Etiology Infection (cytomegalovirus, rubella), subependymal hemorrhage, metabolic diseases, chromosomal deletions (delq6, delp4), cocaine exposure and others.

Pathogenesis Cystic cavity is lined by a pseudocapsule, consisting of aggregates of germinal cells and glial tissue, but no epithelium can be found. Origin of pseudocysts is uncertain. Maybe cystic matrix regression or germinolysis.

Associated anomalies Congenital infection such as cytomegalovirus, congenital heart diseases and associated CNS abnormalities.

Prenatal diagnosis Figures 7.1–7.4.

Differential diagnosis Periventricular leukomalacia.

Prognosis Good in cases with isolated subependymal pseudocysts. In cases with accompanying abnormalities,

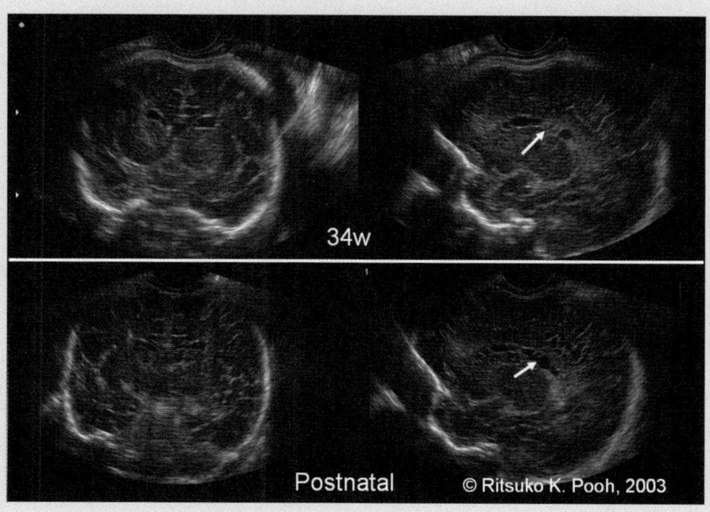

Figure 7.1 Fetal and neonatal ultrasound images of subependymal cysts. Upper, fetal ultrasound images at 34 weeks of gestation. Cystic formation can be observed. Lower, neonatal ultrasound images. The cystic formation has progressed in the echogenic lesion observed *in utero* (arrow). Compare the sagittal section of the fetal and the neonatal images

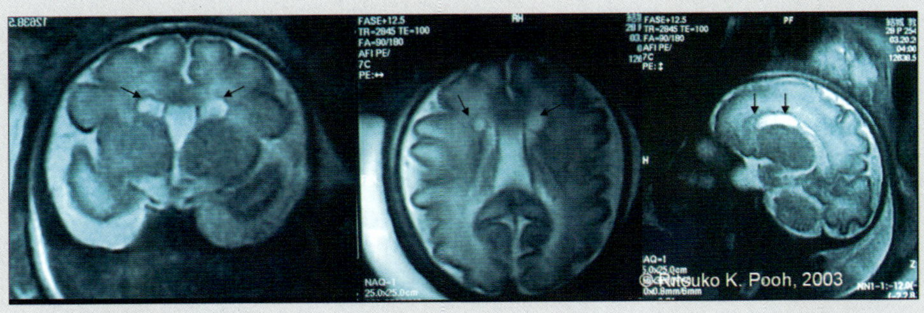

Figure 7.2 Fetal magnetic resonance images of subependymal cysts (same case as shown in Figure 7.1). Bilateral cystic formations (arrows) can be seen in coronal, axial and sagittal images from the left side

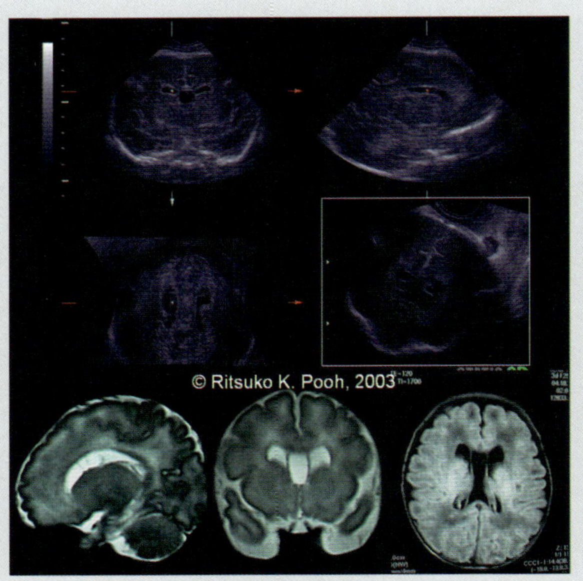

Figure 7.3 Subependymal cysts (fetal ultrasound images and neonatal magnetic resonance images). Upper, coronal and sagittal images. Middle left, axial image. Middle right, anterior coronal section. Note bilateral bead-like cyst formation. Lower, magnetic resonance sagittal, coronal and axial images at 3 days after birth. No neurological symptoms were present at the age of 1 year

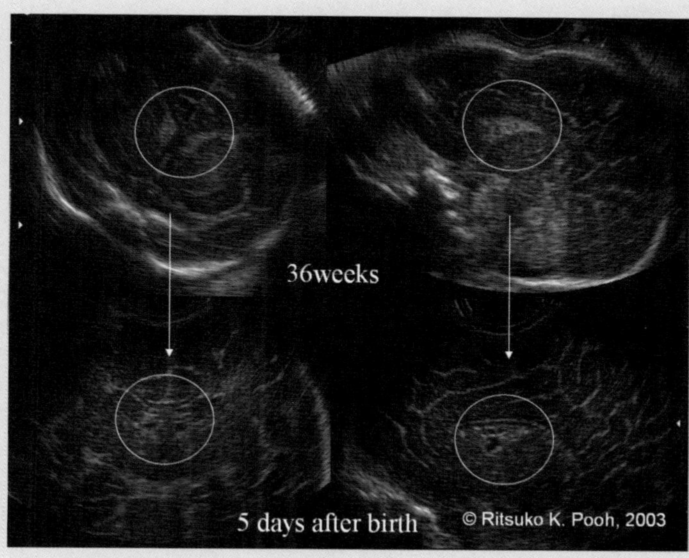

Figure 7.4 Fetal subependymal hemorrhage and cystic formation. Upper left, coronal image at 36 weeks. Upper right, sagittal image at 36 weeks. Lower left, coronal image at day 5 after birth. Lower right, sagittal image at day 5 after birth. Inside bilateral echogenic areas which may indicate hemorrhage, small cysts gradually appeared for a few weeks

such as cardiac disease, cytomegalovirus infection, other intracranial abnormalities, or cases with atypical pseudocysts, prognosis may be poor[1–3].

Recurrence risk Unknown.

Management In many cases, cysts regress during the months after birth. Normal obstetric/neonatal care.

INTRACRANIAL HEMORRHAGE

Incidence Unknown, rare *in utero*.

Definition Hemorrhage, bleeding inside the cranium. Intracranial hemorrhage includes subdural hemorrhage (see Subdural hemorrhage), primary subarachnoid hemorrhage, intracerebellar hemorrhage, intraventricular hemorrhage and intraparenchymal hemorrhage other than cerebellar.

Etiology Trauma, alloimmune and idiopathic thrombocytopenia, von Willebrand's disease, specific medications (warfarin) or illicit drug (cocaine) abuse, seizure, fetal conditions including congenital factor-X and factor-V deficiencies, intracranial tumor, twin–twin transfusion, demise of a co-twin, vascular diseases, or fetomaternal hemorrhage or extracorporeal membrane oxygenation (ECMO)[4,5].

Associated anomalies Hydrocephalus, hydranencephaly, porencephaly or microcephaly.

Prenatal diagnosis Figures 7.5–7.8.

Differential diagnosis Intracranial tumor.

Prognosis Poor in premature infants. Apnea, seizures and other neurological symptoms.

Recurrence risk Depends on etiology.

Management Ventriculoperitoneal shunt if hydrocephalus progresses.

PORENCEPHALY

Incidence Unknown.

Definition Fluid-filled spaces replacing normal brain parenchyma and may or may not communicate with the lateral ventricles or subarachnoid space (Figure 7.9).

Synonym Porencephalic cyst.

Etiology Ischemic episode, trauma[6], demise of one twin, intercerebral hemorrhage and infection.

Pathogenesis Occurs when the immature cerebrum has some factors with propensity for dissolution and cavitation (e.g. high content of water, myelinated fiber bundles, deficient astroglial response). The timing of ischemic injury (maybe as early as the second trimester) is strongly related to porencephaly and hydranencephaly[7].

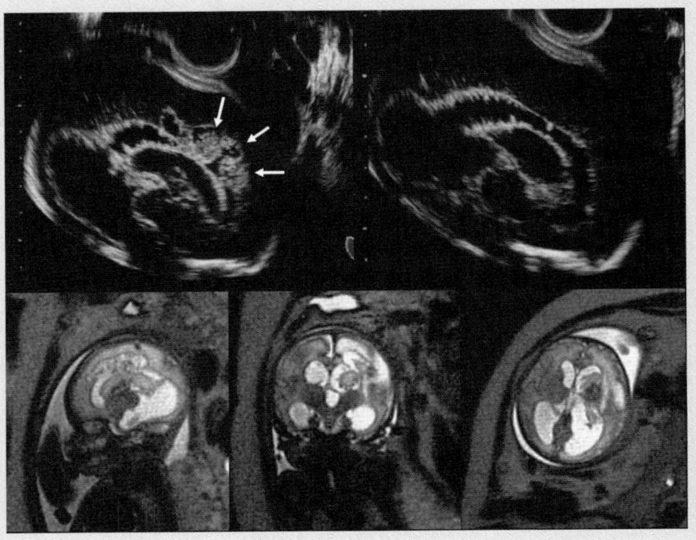

Figure 7.5 Intracerebral/intraventricular hemorrhage during pregnancy. Upper, ultrasound at 32 weeks; lower, fetal magnetic resonance image at 33 weeks. No maternal traumatic and/or bleeding episode occurred. Upper left, sagittal ultrasound image of ventriculomegaly and a high-echogenic periventricular hemorrhage (arrows). Echogenicity of the inside wall of the ventricle indicates an intraventricular hemorrhage. Upper right, the other ventricle. No periventricular hemorrhage, but an intraventricular hemorrhage can be seen. Lower, fetal magnetic resonance images. Images courtesy of Dr T. Murakoshi

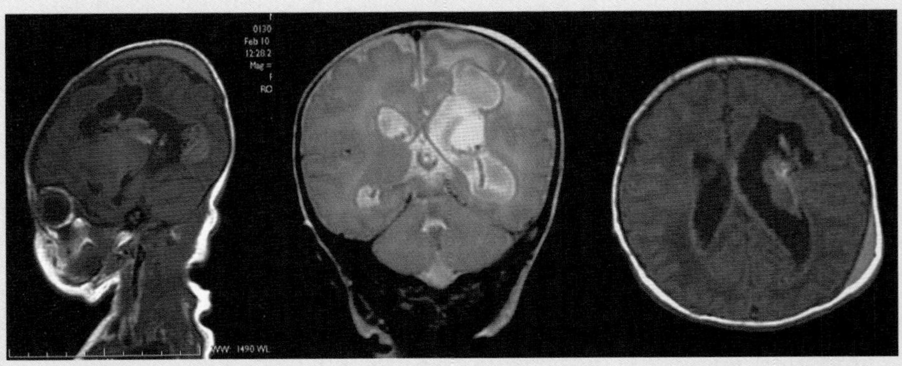

Figure 7.6 Postnatal magnetic resonance image (same case as shown in Figure 7.5). Left, sagittal section. Middle, coronal section. Right, axial section. Porencephalic change in the hemorrhagic lesion is demonstrated. (See 'Porencephaly' in this Chapter). Images courtesy of Dr T. Murakoshi

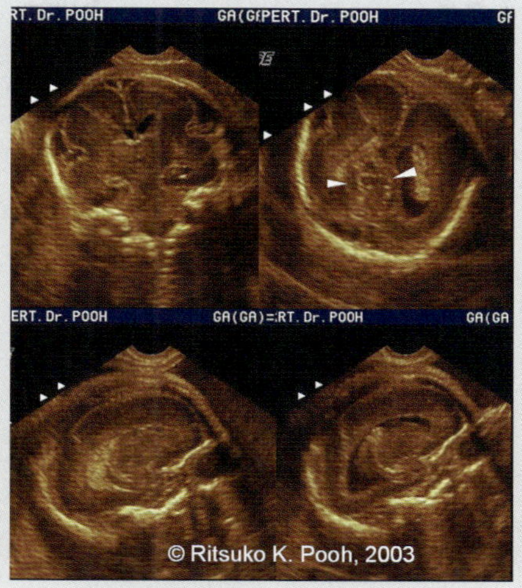

Figure 7.7 A unilateral slit-like ventricle due to an intracranial hemorrhage (24 weeks of gestation). Upper left, coronal anterior section. There is a conspicuous difference between the anterior horns of the ventricles. Upper right, coronal posterior section. Note the asymmetrical hemisphere and intracranial hemorrhage (arrowheads). Lower, parasagittal section of each lateral ventricle. A unilateral slit-like ventricle (no space inside the ventricle but in the choroid plexus) is clearly demonstrated. This is different from ventricular asymmetry of a normal variation. The hemorrhage and slit ventricle spontaneously resolved and the case had a normal postnatal course for 2 years. Postnatal magnetic resonance imaging shows mild ventricular asymmetry of normal variation

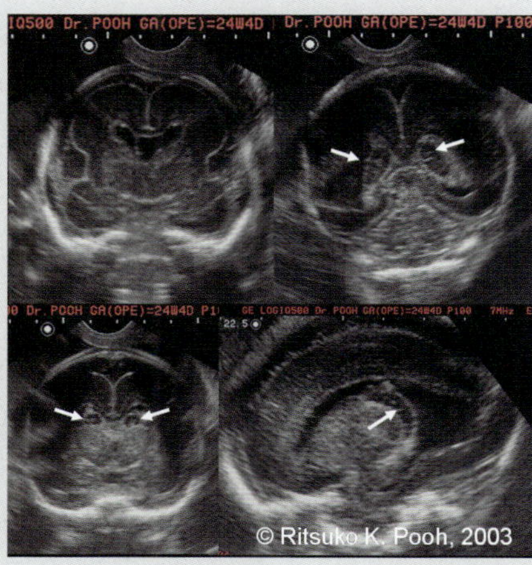

Figure 7.8 Intraventricular hemorrhage (24 weeks of gestation). A transvaginal scan from an early stage showing normal imaging until 20 weeks. From 22 weeks, mild ventriculomegaly and bilateral hemorrhage inside the choroid plexus (arrows) could be seen. The lesion is differentiated from a choroid plexus cyst by echogenicity. In this case, the hemorrhage spontaneously disappeared by 30 weeks, with a normal magnetic resonance image after birth and no neurological deficit seen at the age of 2 years

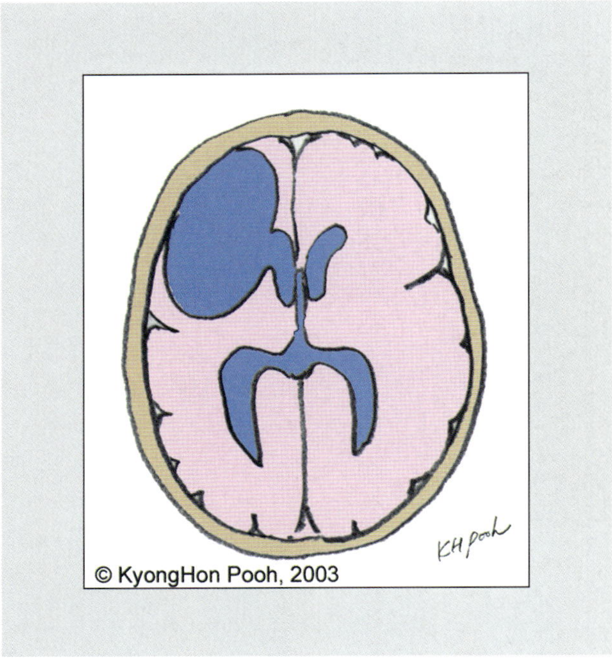

Figure 7.9 Schematic representation of porencephaly. Porencephaly is a single unilateral cavity within the cerebral hemishpere that may or may not be communicated by the lateral ventricle. Causes of porencephaly include ischemia, intracerebral hemorrhage or infection. A porencephalic cyst never causes a mass effect, which is observed in cases with an arachnoid cyst or other cystic mass lesions. This condition is an acquired brain insult and is differentiated from schizencephaly of migration disorder

Associated anomalies Intercerebral hemorrhage, interventricular hemorrhage and hydrocephalus.

Prenatal diagnosis Figure 7.10. Some cases *in utero* have been reported[8,9].

Differential diagnosis Schizencephaly, arachnoid cyst, intracranial cystic tumor and other cysts. Porencephalic cysts never cause a mass effect, which is observed in cases with an arachnoid cyst or other cystic mass lesions. This condition is an acquired brain insult and is differentiated from schizencephaly of migration disorder.

Prognosis Various, depends on timing and size of the lesion. Seizures, neurological deficits and cerebral palsy often occur[10].

Recurrence risk Unknown.

Management Ventriculoperitoneal shunt if hydrocephalus progresses (Figure 7.11).

HYDRANENCEPHALY

Incidence 1–2.5/10000 births.

Definition Absence of the cerebral hemispheres and a sac-like structure containing cerebral spinal fluid surrounding the brainstem and basal ganglia.

Etiology Ischemic episode, trauma, demise of one twin, intercerebral hemorrhage and infection. There

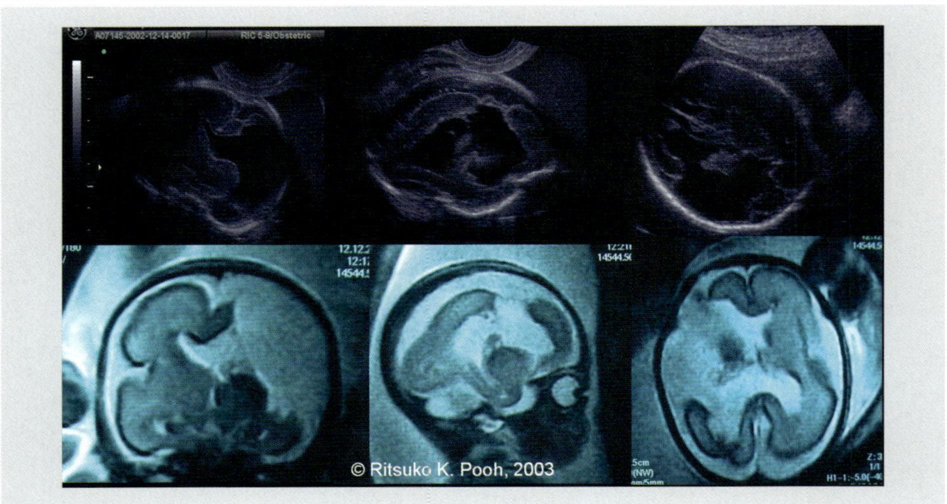

Figure 7.10 Fetal ultrasound and magnetic resonance images of porencephaly at 25 weeks of gestation. Upper left, transvaginal ultrasound coronal image. Defect of the parietolateral part of the unilateral cerebrum. This case also has an absent septum pellucidum. Upper middle, parasagittal ultrasound image. The porencephalic area connects to the unilateral ventricle. Echogenicity of the inside of the ventricular wall indicates an intraventricular hemorrhage. Upper right, transabdominal ultrasound axial image. Lower, fetal magnetic resonance images on the same day; coronal, parasagittal and axial sections from the left side

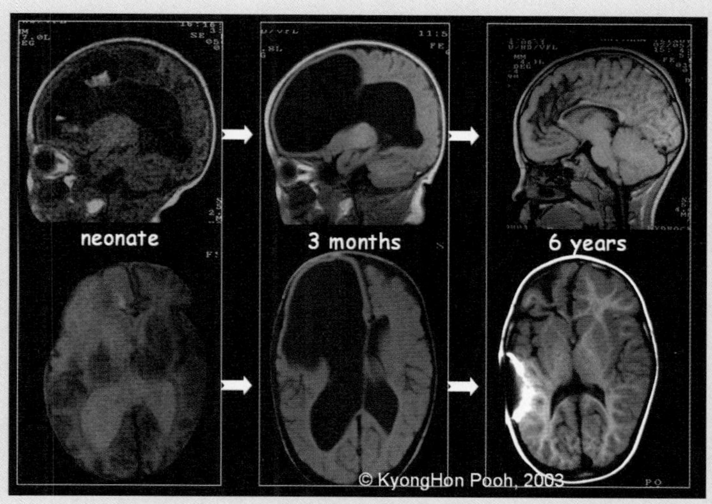

Figure 7.11 Treatment of porencephaly. Left, neonatal magnetic resonance images. Frontal porencephaly fused with moderately enlarged ventricle is demonstrated. Middle, magnetic resonance images 3 months after birth. Enlargement of a porencephalic cyst and the ventricles is demonstrated. A ventriculo-peritoneal shunt was placed due to progressive hydrocephalus. Right, magnetic resonance images at the age of 6 years demonstrating disappeared porencephalic cyst and a developed cerebrum instead

are several theories but bilateral occlusion of the supraclinoid segment of the internal carotid arteries[11] or of the middle cerebral arteries is one of the causes of subtotal defects of the cerebral hemisphere.

Pathogenesis Occurs when the immature cerebrum has some factors with propensity for dissolution and cavitation (e.g. high content of water, myelinated fiber bundles, deficient astroglial response). The timing of ischemic injury (maybe as early as the second trimester) is strongly related to porencephaly and hydranencephaly. Recently, hydranencephaly from 11 weeks of gestation has been reported[12].

Associated anomalies Large head (Figure 7.12).

Differential diagnosis Massive hydrocephalus, alobar holoprosencephaly, porencephaly.

Prognosis Extremely poor.

Recurrence risk Unknown.

Management No active treatment. Shunt procedure for progressive increase of infant's head.

SUBDURAL HEMORRHAGE

Incidence Rare (extremely rare in fetuses).

Definition Blood or coagula collection between the dura mater and the arachnoid membrane (Figure 7.13).

Synonyms Subdural hematoma.

Etiology *In utero* trauma, maternal thrombocytopenia[13] (immune, alloimmune, idiopathic), traumatic deliveries and unknown causes.

Pathogenesis Hemorrhage from subdural blood vessels by defective coagulation or trauma.

Associated anomalies Fracture or decompression of the skull, porencephaly, hydrocephalus, hydrops, tentorial laceration, falx laceration and cerebral convexity.

Prenatal diagnosis Figure 7.14.

Differential diagnosis Intracranial hemorrhage in another location or intracranial tumor.

Prognosis Infants with a major tentorial/falx laceration with massive hemorrhage have a very poor prognosis. Fetal demise, neonatal demise, or neurological deficits of seizures, hypotonia and severe mental retardation[14–17]. However, cases with subdural hematomas in the posterior fossa have a favorable prognosis even without surgical treatment.

Recurrence risk Depends on the causes of the hemorrhage. There is a high recurrence rate with alloimmune thrombocytopenia.

Management Timing of delivery and mode of delivery should be considered. Neurosurgical intervention is not always necessary when the infant is stable

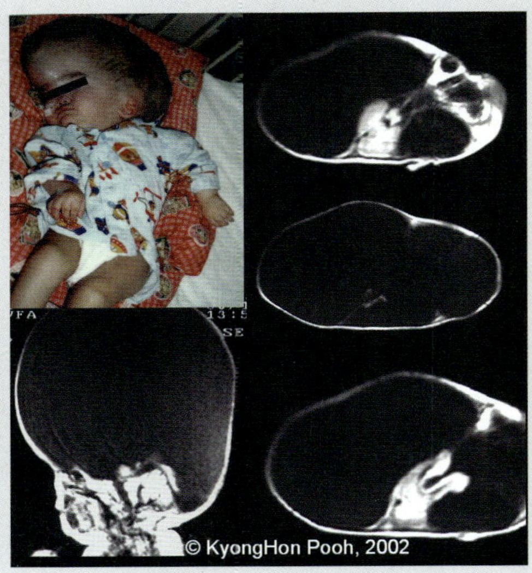

Figure 7.12 Hydranencephaly is characterized by the absence of the cerebral hemispheres with an incomplete or absent falx and a sac-like structure containing cerebral spinal fluid surrounding the brainstem and basal ganglia. In this case, tentorium and falx cerebri are recognized. The cerebral cortex is depicted in only a small part of the occipital lobe. The brainstem and cerebellum are preserved as normal. The cause of the hydranencephaly may be obstruction of the bilateral internal carotid arteries. Note the remarkable increase in the head circumference

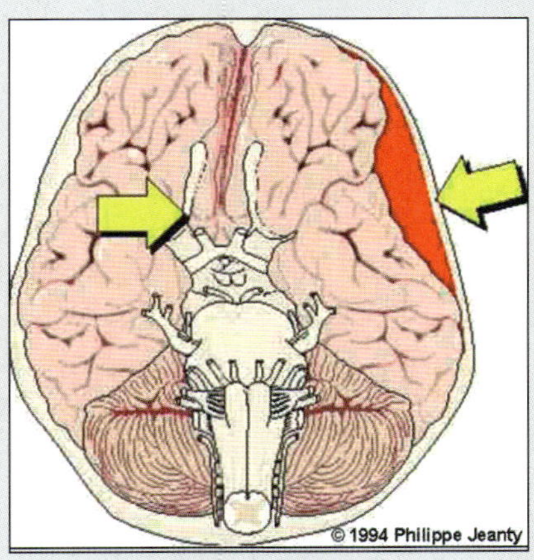

Figure 7.13 Subdural hemorrhage (in red) assumes a lenticular shape between the hard skull and the depressed brain. Schema courtesy of Dr P. Jeanty, www.TheFetus.net, with permission

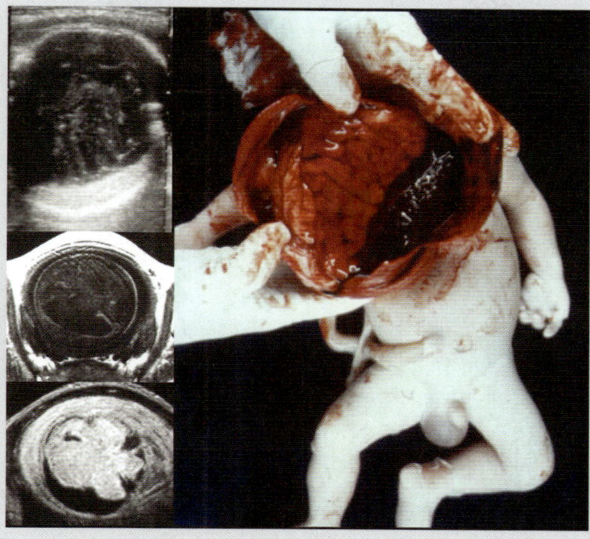

Figure 7.14 Fetal subdural hematoma. Upper left, antenatal sonographic image. The bright echogenic area indicates a hemorrhage. Middle left, fetal magnetic resonance (T1) image. Lower left, fetal magnetic resonance (T2) image. Right, photograph of stillborn infant. Images and photograph courtesy of Dr I. Kawabata

neurologically. When neurological deficits are manifest, subdural taps can be done.

POLYMICROGYRIA (POSTMIGRATIONAL POLYMICROGYRIA)

Incidence Unknown, very rare.

Definition A great number of small placations in the cortical surface, rendering to the external aspect of the cerebrum the appearance of a wrinkled chestnut. There are two basic varieties of polymicrogyria:

(1) *Layered* Postmigrational and related to destructive process;

(2) *Unlayered* Neuronal migrational disorder, accompanied by another migration disorder.

In this Chapter, layered polymicrogyria due to postmigrational causes is considered.

Etiology Ischemic encephaloclastic mechanism[18], maldevelopment, cytomegalovirus infection[19].

Pathogenesis Laminar neuronal necrosis in the cortex after the apparent completion of migration.

Associated anomalies Periventricular leukomalacia[18].

Prenatal diagnosis Figures 7.15–7.18.

Prognosis Neurological development is often severely deranged.

Recurrence risk Unknown.

Management Standard obstetric and neonatal care.

FETAL PERIVENTRICULAR LEUKOMALACIA

Incidence 25–75% of premature infants at autopsy have complications of periventricular white matter injury. However, clinically, incidence may be much lower. Five to 10% of infants have a birth weight of less than 1500 g. In term infants, periventricular leukomalacia (PVL) is very rare.

Definition Multifocal areas of necrosis are found deep in the cortical white matter, which are often symmetrical and occur adjacent to the lateral ventricles. PVL represents a major precursor for neurological and intellectual impairment, and cerebral palsy in later life.

Etiology Birth trauma, asphyxia and respiratory failure, cardiopulmonary defects, premature birth/low birth weight, associated immature cerebrovascular development and lack of appropriate autoregulation of cerebral blood flow in response to hypoxic–ischemic insults[20].

Pathogenesis Distinctive and consists primarily of both focal periventricular necrosis and more diffuse

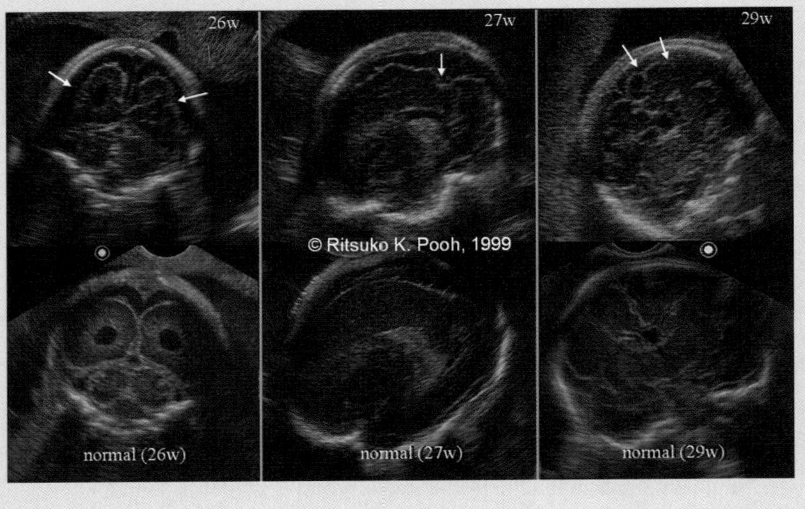

Figure 7.15 Atrophic brain with polymicrogyria at 26–29 weeks of gestation. The lower images are normal brain images at the same gestational age. Brain atrophy became conspicuous (arrows) from 25 weeks (3 weeks after an ischemic episode). Left, posterior coronal section at 26 weeks. Middle, parasagittal section at 27 weeks. Right, anterior coronal section at 29 weeks. Note the polymicrogyral formation in the parietofrontal area. This condition is referred to as postmigrational polymicrogyria

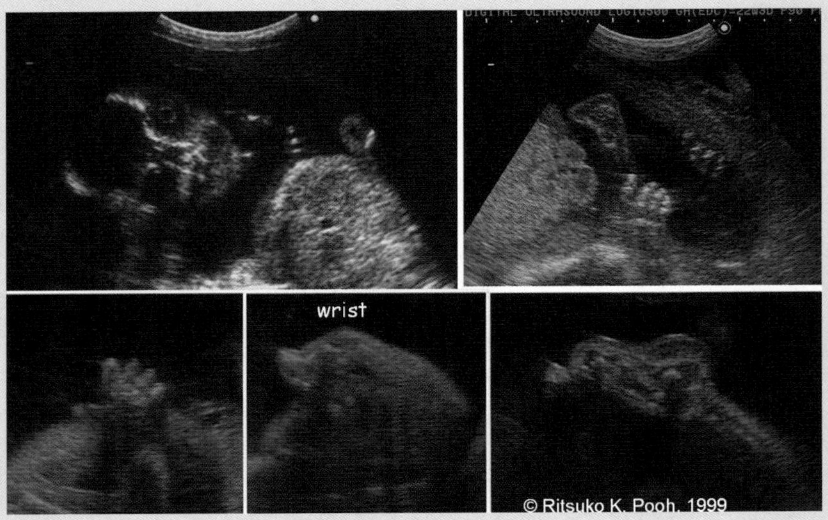

Figure 7.16 Fetal akinetic phase after an ischemic episode (upper) and hypertonic phase 3 weeks later (lower; same fetus as shown in Figure 7.15). A fetal ischemic–hypoxic episode associated with maternal shock state due to an unknown cause occurred at 22 weeks. No fetal movements except heart beats were observed for 5 days after the episode (upper). After 5 days of akinetic phase, the fetal extremities became hypertonic and contractural (lower). However, the fetus moved actively *in utero* with hypertonic hands and feet

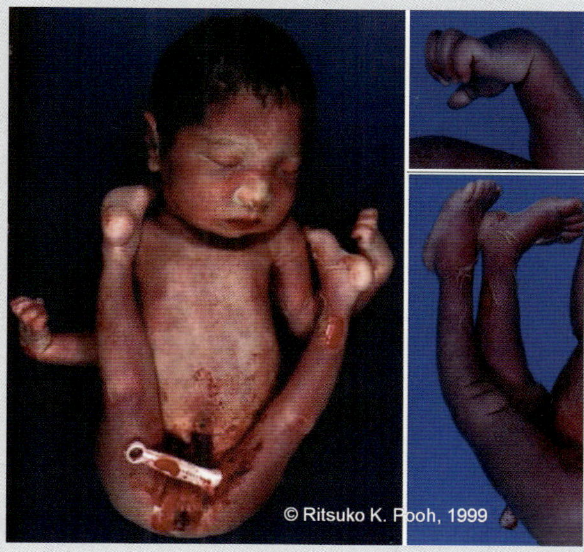

Figure 7.17 External appearance of a stillborn fetus at 31 weeks of gestation (same case as shown in Figures 7.15 and 7.16). Left, stillborn fetus. Sudden intrauterine fetal demise occurred at 31 weeks of gestation. Right, extremities. Hypertonic and contractural appearance of the extremities is quite similar to the fetal appearance *in utero* as shown in Figure 7.16

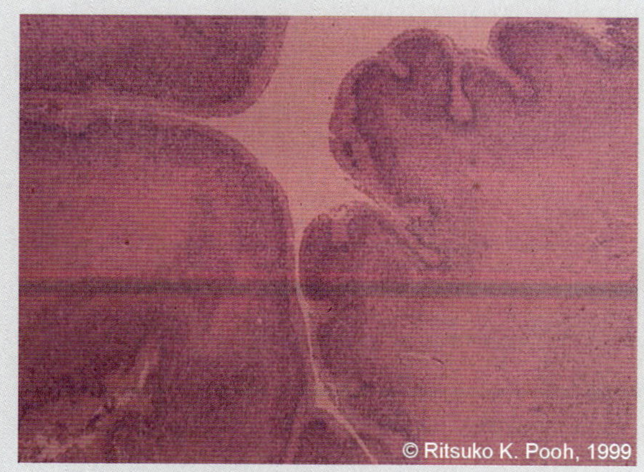

Figure 7.18 Polymicrogyria in the same case as shown in Figures 7.15–7.17. Polymicrogyria is demonstrated due to an ischemic and hypoxic episode at 22 weeks of gestation. Postmigrational polymicrogyria

cerebral white matter injury. The two most common sites are at the level of the cerebral white matter near the trigone of the lateral ventricles and around the foramen of Monro. Volpe[21] describes three factors, strongly related to PVL:

(1) Periventricular vascular anatomical and physiological factors;

(2) Cerebral ischemia;

(3) Intrinsic vulnerability of the cerebral white matter of premature newborns.

Prenatal diagnosis Figures 7.19–7.21.

Differential diagnosis Subarachnoid (periventricular) pseudocysts, porencephaly and other intracranial cystic formations.

Prognosis A neurological feature of PVL in the neonatal period is probable lower limb weakness and features such as long-term sequelae, spastic diplegia, intellectual deficits and visual deficits are observed[21].

Recurrence risk Unknown.

Management Early rehabilitation.

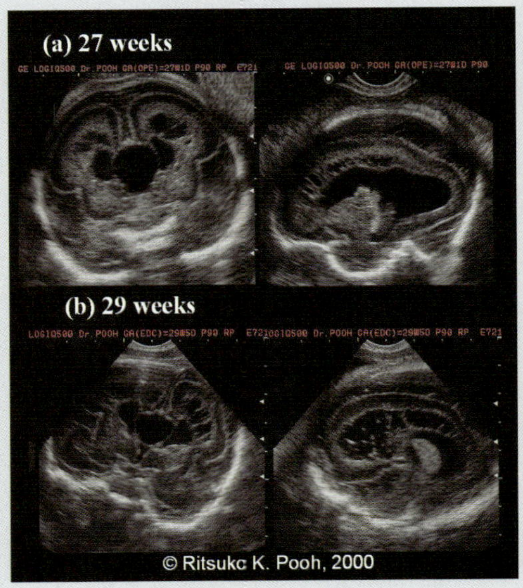

Figure 7.19 Fetal periventricular leukomalacia (PVL). (a) Fetal ultrasound at 27 weeks. Clear bilateral PVL is observed with mild ventriculomegaly and enlargement of the cavum septum pellucidum. (b) 29 weeks, PVL was progressive and became widespread

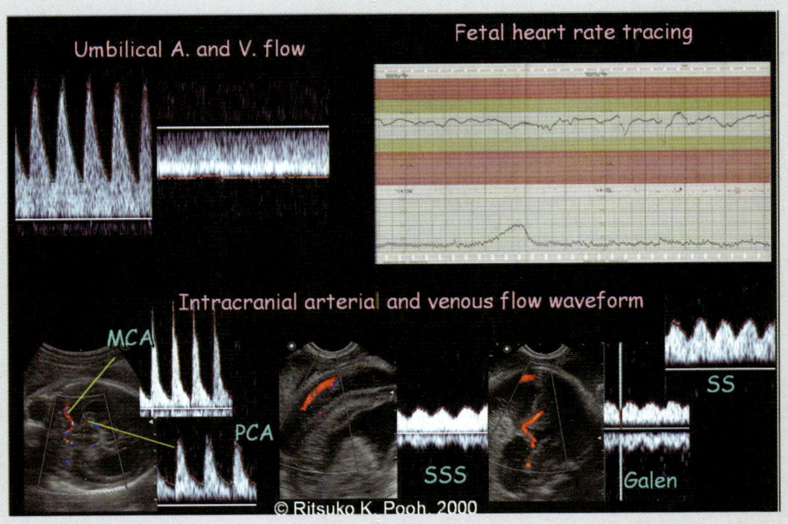

Figure 7.20 Flow waveforms and fetal heart rate tracing at 27 weeks of gestation in a case of PVL (same case as shown in Figure 7.19). Upper left, umbilical arterial and venous flow – normal circulation. Upper right, fetal heart rate tracing. Normal reactivity is demonstrated. Lower, intracranial arterial and venous flow waveforms. Blood flow waveforms of the middle cerebral artery (MCA), posterior cerebral artery (PCA), superior sagittal sinus (SSS), vein of Galen (Galen) and straight sinus (SS) are all normal

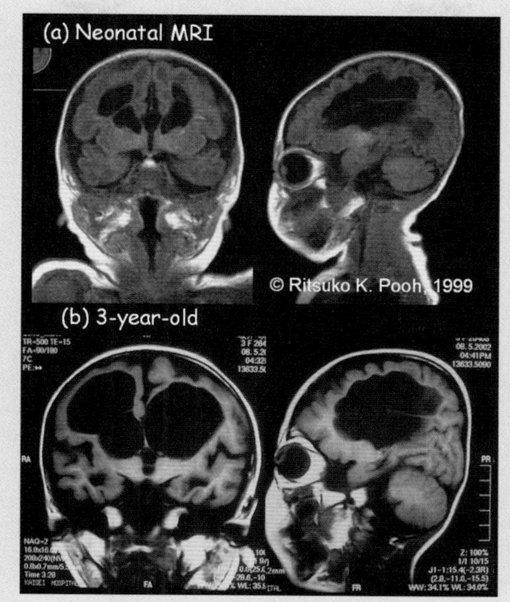

Figure 7.21 Periventricular leukomalacia (PVL) (same case as shown in Figures 7.18 and 7.19). (a) Neonatal magnetic resonance image. Widespread type of PVL is clear. (b) Magnetic resonance image at the age of 3 years. The PVL lesion completely changed into a 'defect of the cerebrum'. Early rehabilitation training started from the neonatal stage because of prenatal detection of PVL. Severe cerebral palsy was seen with spastic quadriplegia. Magnetic resonance images at age of 3 years, courtesy of Dr K. Fukuda

FETAL PERIVENTRICULAR ECHODENSITY

Incidence Infrequent but not rare in clinically high-risk fetuses.

Definition Periventricular echodensity (PVE) is a highly echogenic periventricular image, of which echogenicity is higher than the choriod plexus in the visual analysis of the ultrasonic brain image.

Etiology It is thought to be caused by a hypoxic–ischemic lesion of the fetal brain, which may be the same as neonatal PVL, and is estimated to be at the lightest end of its spectrum.

Pathogenesis Simple PVE does not result in fetal death. It can progress into neonatal PVL, if it persists until birth, particularly in a preterm infant.

Prenatal diagnosis Figures 7.22–7.25.

Prognosis Neonatal PVL followed by cerebral palsy (CP) can occur in fetal PVE which persists until delivery, especially in preterm birth. The CP ratio is higher in the fetus whose PVE persists until the birth, than in the fetus who has no PVE, or whose PVE disappeared before birth, and is higher than the common CP incidence (Table 7.1).

Management Prevention of preterm delivery particularly in high-risk fetuses who have suffered cord complications and preterm labor. Careful ultrasonic study of the brain is needed in neonates who suffer PVE before birth, particularly when it persists until delivery.

BRAIN TUMORS

Incidence Extremely rare.

Definition Tumors located in the intracranial cavity.

Histological types Brain tumors are divided into teratomas, most commonly reported, and non-teratomatous tumors. Non-teratomatous tumors include neuroepithelial tumors, such as medulloblastoma, astrocytoma, choroid plexus papilloma, choroid plexus carcinoma, ependymoma, ependymoblastoma; mesenchymal tumors such as craniopharyngioma, sarcoma, fibroma, hemangioblastoma, hemangioma and meningoma; and other tumors such as lipoma of the corpus callosum, and subependymal giant-cell astrocytoma associated with tuberous sclerosis (often accompanied by cardiac rhabdomyoma)[24,25].

Location of tumor Supratentorial predominance in neonatal tumors; infratentorial predominance in medulloblastoma. Choroid plexus papilloma is located within the lateral ventricles.

Associated abnormalities Macrocrania or local skull swelling, epignathus, secondary hydrocephalus, intracranial hemorrhage, intraventricular hemorrhage, polyhydramnios, heart failure by high cardiac output[26] and hydrops.

Table 7.1 Neonatal periventricular leukomalacia (PVL) and cerebral palsy (CP) are frequent in the cases of persistent fetal periventricular echogenicity (PVE) until the birth, particularly in preterm cases, whereas no PVL or CP appeared among the cases of no PVE or those of disappeared PVE before the birth [2]. The pathological nature of the fetal PVE is estimated from the results

Outcome	*No fetal PVE*	*Disappeared PVE before birth*	*Persistent PVE until birth*	*Fetal PVE (b + c)*	*Total (a + b + c)*
Normal	21 (a)	19 (b)	23 (c)	42 (b + c)	63
Neonatal PVL	0	0	5/23 (21.7%)*	5/42 (11.9%)	5
CP	0	0	4/23 (17.4%)†	4/42 (9.5%)‡	4

Four preterm and one term births are included in five cases of PVL out of 23 persistent PVE cases.
†Four CP are included in the five PVL; PVL (21.7%)* and CP (17.4%)† occur more frequently in the 23 persistent cases of PVE than both (0%) do in cases with no PVE and disappeared PVE; ‡CP ratio (9.5%) is higher in the 42 cases of fetal PVE than the common CP ratio (0.2%)

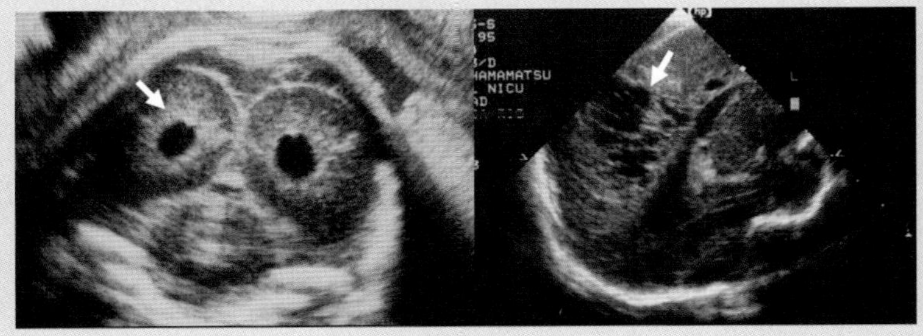

Figure 7.22 A case of fetal periventricular echogenicity (PVE) with high echogenicity that is as bright as the choroid plexus, or more echogenic, and its gray-level histogram width (GLHW) value is higher than that for a normal brain (see Chapter 3)[23]. The case was a large baby of monochorionic twins, whose PVE (white arrow, left panel) was recorded in the posterior coronal section[22] with transvaginal sonography at 28 weeks of pregnancy. The PVE persisted until the birth at 30 weeks. The neonate developed PVL, and its typical change was recorded at 25 days (white arrow, right panel). Cerebral palsy was confirmed at 2 years[23]. Image courtesy of Dr N. Yamamoto, Dr M. Utsu and Dr T. Murakoshi

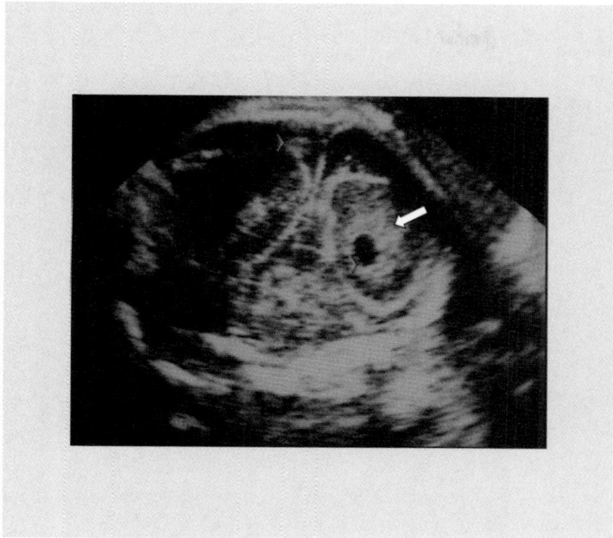

Figure 7.23 Fetal periventricular echogenicity (PVE) (arrow) was recorded in the posterior coronal section[22] with transvaginal sonography at 29 weeks of pregnancy. Fetal pulmonary sequestration and polyhydramnios were also detected. The PVE persisted until birth at 32 weeks. Cystic periventricular leukomalacia was found on day 14. Cerebral palsy was confirmed at 1 year[23]. Image courtesy of Dr N. Yamamoto, Dr M. Utsu and Dr T. Murakoshi

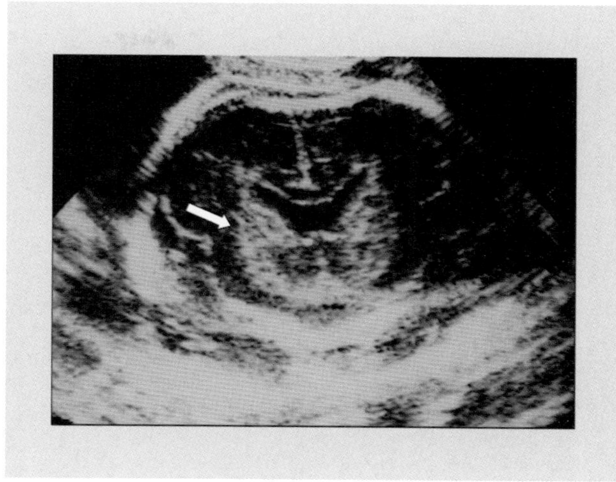

Figure 7.24 The periventricular echogenicity (PVE) (arrow) was recorded in median coronal section[22] with transvaginal sonography at 27 weeks of pregnancy in a case of premature labor. The PVE persisted until the birth under tocolysis with β-mimetics due to the contractions. A premature female baby was born at 28 weeks without diminution of the PVE which was also found in the neonatal brain. Cystic periventricular leukomalacia and spastic paraplegia appeared afterwards[23]. Image courtesy of Dr N. Yamamoto, Dr M. Utsu and Dr T. Murakoshi

Diagnosis Intracranial masses with solid, cystic or mixed pattern with or without visualization of hypervascularity by ultrasound and fetal MRI. A brain tumor should be considered in cases with unexplained intracranial hemorrhage.

Prenatal diagnosis Figures 7.26–7.31.

Differential diagnosis Arachnoid cyst, vein of Galen aneurysm, porencephaly, schizencephaly, periventricular leukomalacia and subdural hemorrhage.

Prognosis Fetal demise; stillbirth may occur. Prognosis in neonates is generally poor, but depends on timing of diagnosis and the histological type of tumor. Choroid plexus papilloma has minimal mortality rate and a high likelihood of good neonatal outcome. The mortality rate for teratomas is over 90% and for medulloblastoma over 80%. Other tumors have various prognoses.

Recurrence risk Unknown.

Management Cesarean section may be considered. Neurosurgical tumor resection including subtotal hemispherectomy by craniotomy and chemotherapy are possible treatments for neonatal tumors. Radiation therapy is usually not indicated in neonates.

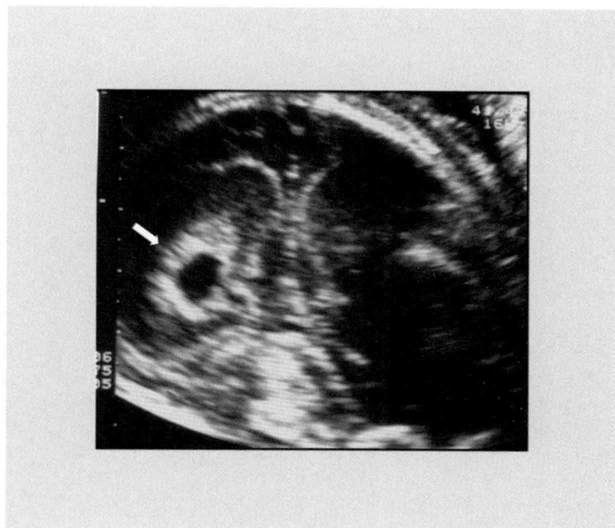

Figure 7.25 Fetal periventricular echogenicity (PVE) (arrow) was recorded in the posterior coronal section[22] with transvaginal sonography at 29 weeks of pregnancy in a case of preterm labor and subependymal hemorrhage (SEH). The PVE persisted until birth at 37 weeks. Bilateral SEH and PVE were confirmed on day 2 and a small cystic periventricular leukomalacia on day 11. No neurological abnormality was found at 3 years[23]. Image courtesy of Dr N. Yamamoto, Dr M. Utsu and Dr T. Murakoshi

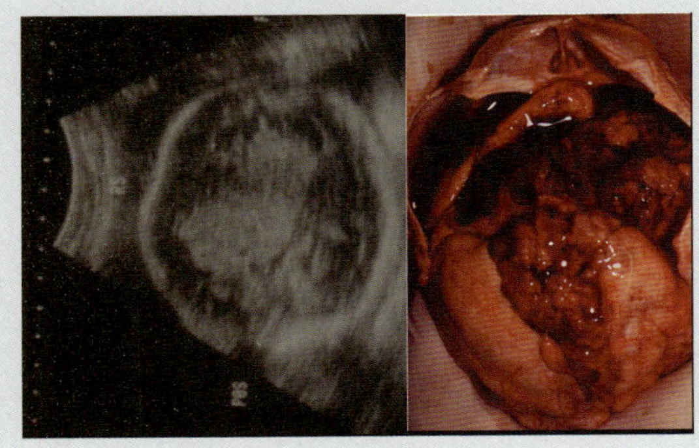

Figure 7.26 Immature teratoma. Left, high echogenic huge brain mass at 30 weeks of gestation. Right, autopsy finding of huge tumor. Immature teratoma was confirmed histologically. Image and photograph courtesy of Dr M. Utsu

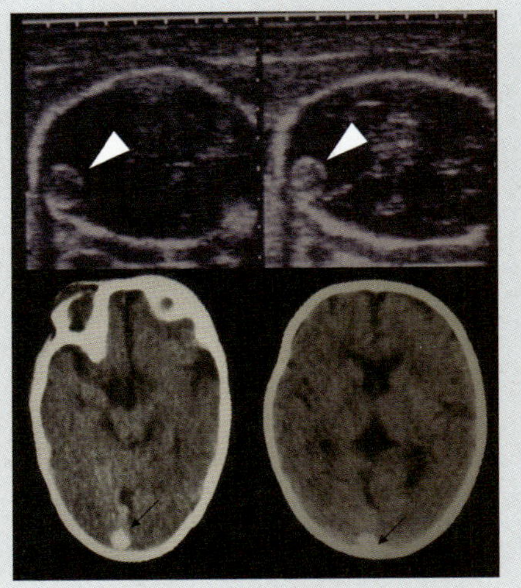

Figure 7.27 Mature teratoma. Upper, prenatal ultrasound at 28 weeks of gestation. A clear high echogenic lesion is demonstrated (arrowhead). Lower, postnatal CT axial image. Images courtesy of Dr M. Utsu

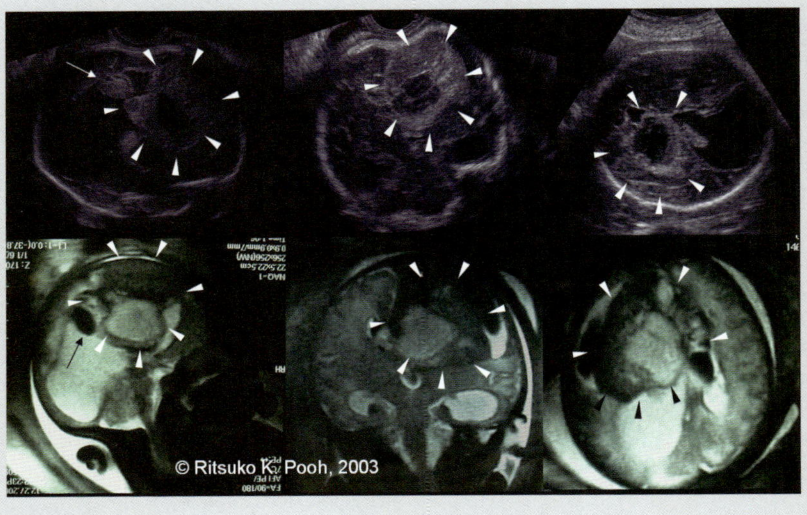

Figure 7.28 Fetal ultrasound and magnetic resonance imaging of a brain tumor with tumoral and interventricular hemorrhage (35 weeks and 5 days of gestation). Upper, sagittal, coronal and axial ultrasound images. A huge tumor (arrowheads) with a hemorrhage within the tumor in the frontoparietal lobe is complicated by unilateral hydrocephalus with an intraventricular hemorrhage (arrow). Lower, sagittal, coronal and axial magnetic resonance images

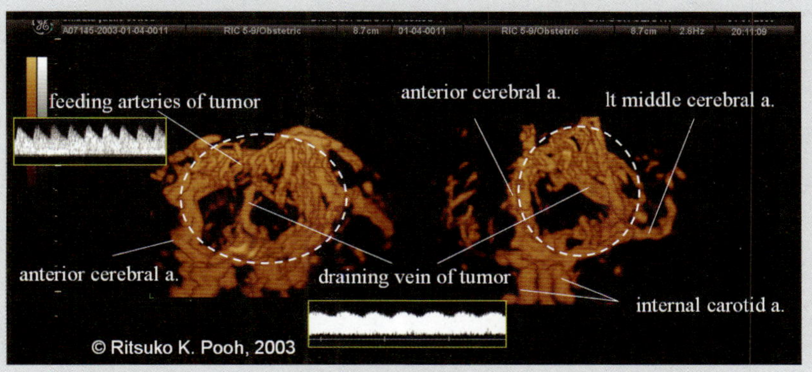

Figure 7.29 Tumoral vascular visualization by three-dimensional power Doppler (same case as shown in Figure 7.28). Left, oblique sagittal view from fetal left side. Right, oblique coronal view from fetal frontal side. The tumor is fed by numerous feeding arteries from the anterior cerebral artery. Feeder arteries have a low resistant flow waveform. One large vein which drains blood from the tumor is visible. The draining vein has flow pulsation

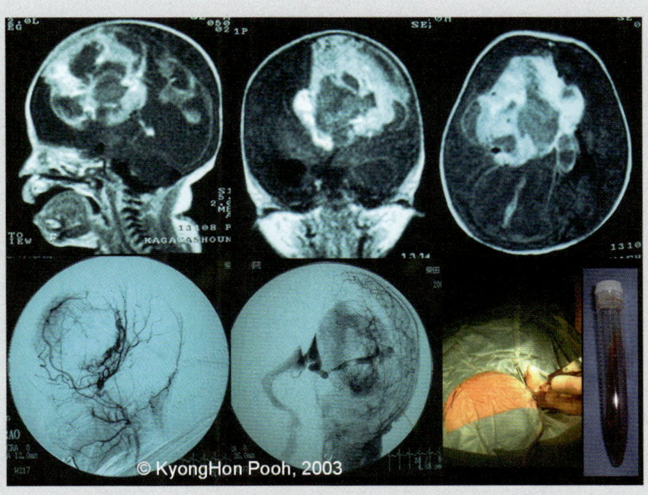

Figure 7.30 Postnatal magnetic resonance image (MRI), angiography and drained fluid from ventricle (same case as shown in Figures 7.28 and 7.29). A female 2950-g baby was delivered by Cesarean section with an Apgar score of 8. Upper, magnetic resonance T1-weighted images after birth. Note intensity of the enlarged left ventricle which indicates intraventricular blood collection. Lower left and middle, sagittal and coronal angiography. Arterial phase (left) shows feeding arteries from the anterior cerebral artery. Venous phase (middle) shows draining vein and tumor stain. Lower right, drainage of intraventricular hemorrhagic fluid through a miniature Ommaya reservoir. At the 10th postnatal day, a tumor resection by craniotomy was successfully performed and the postoperative course has been good

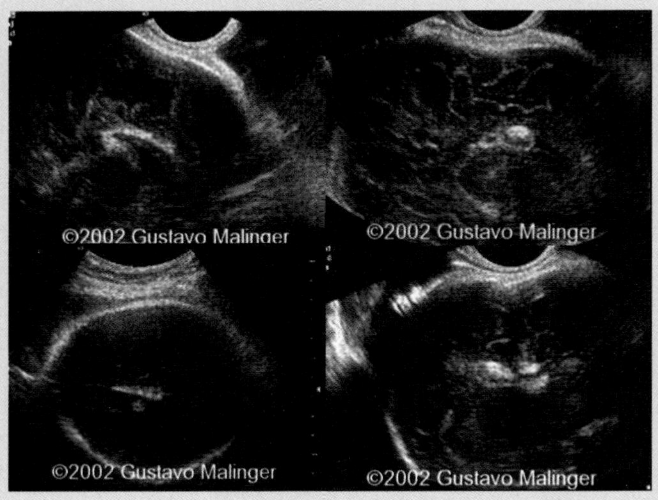

Figure 7.31 Lipoma of the corpus callosum. The pregnancy had been followed by serial ultrasound examination because of mild ventriculomegaly since the 23rd week of gestation. Upper, sagittal sections. Lower left, axial section. Lower right, coronal section. Note the pericallosal high echogenicity. Images courtesy of Dr G. Malinger, www.TheFetus.net, with permission

REFERENCES

1. Lu JH, Emons D, Kowalewski S. Connatal periventricular pseudocysts in the neonate. *Pediatr Radiol* 1992;22:55–8
2. Malinger G, Lev D, Ben Sira L, *et al.* Congenital periventricular pseudocysts: prenatal sonographic appearance and clinical implications. *Ultrasound Obstet Gynecol* 2002;20:447–51
3. Bats AS, Molho M, Senat MV, *et al.* Subependymal pseudocysts in the fetal brain: prenatal diagnosis of two cases and review of the literature. *Ultrasound Obstet Gynecol* 2002;20:502–5
4. Sherer DM, Anyaegbunam A, Onyeije C. Antepartum fetal intracranial hemorrhage, predisposing factors and prenatal sonography: a review. *Am J Perinatol* 1998;15:431–41
5. Hardart GE, Fackler JC. Predictors of intracranial hemorrhage during neonatal extracorporeal membrane oxygenation. *J Pediatr* 1999;134:156–9
6. Eller KM, Kuller JA. Porencephaly secondary to fetal trauma during amniocentesis. *Obstet Gynecol* 1995;85:865–7
7. Volpe JJ. Hypoxic–ischemic encephalopathy: neuropathology and pathogenesis. In *Neurology of the Newborn*. 4th edn. Philadelphia: W.B. Saunders, 2001:296-330
8. Meizner I, Elchalal U. Prenatal sonographic diagnosis of anterior fossa porencephaly. *J Clin Ultrasound* 1996;24:96–9
9. de Laveaucoupet J, Audibert F, Guis F, *et al.* Fetal magnetic resonance imaging (MRI) of ischemic brain injury. *Prenat Diagn* 2001;21:729–36
10. Scher MS, Belfar H, Martin J, *et al.* Destructive brain lesions of presumed fetal onset: antepartum causes of cerebral palsy. *Pediatrics* 1991;88:898–906
11. Stevenson DA, Hart BL, Clericuzio CL. Hydranencephaly in an infant with vascular malformations. *Am J Med Genet* 2001;104:295–8
12. Lam YH, Tang MH. Serial sonographic features of a fetus with hydranencephaly from 11 weeks to term. *Ultrasound Obstet Gynecol* 2000;16:77–9
13. Demir RH, Gleicher N, Myers SA. Atraumatic antepartum subdural hematoma causing fetal death. *Am J Obstet Gynecol* 1989;160:619–20
14. Meagher SE, Walker SP, Choong S. Mid-trimester fetal subdural hemorrhage: prenatal diagnosis. *Ultrasound Obstet Gynecol* 2002;20:296–8

15. Rotmensch S, Grannum PA, Nores JA, *et al.* *In utero* diagnosis and management of fetal subdural hematoma. *Am J Obstet Gynecol* 1991;164:1246–8

16. Gunn TR, Mok PM, Becroft DMO. Subdural hemorrhage *in utero*. *Pediatrics* 1985;76:605–9

17. Bussel JB, Berkowitz RL, McFarland JG, *et al.* Antenatal treatment of neonatal alloimmune thrombocytopenia. *N Engl J Med* 1988;319:1374–8

18. Inder TE, Huppi PS, Zientara GP, *et al.* The post-migrational development of polymicrogyria documented by magnetic resonance imaging from 31 weeks' postconceptional age. *Ann Neurol* 1999;45:798–801

19. Marques Dias MJ, Harmant-van Rijckevorsel G, Landrieu P, *et al.* Prenatal cytomegalovirus disease and cerebral microgyria: evidence for perfusion failure, not disturbance of histogenesis, as the major cause of fetal cytomegalovirus encephalopathy. *Neuropediatrics* 1984;15:18–24

20. Rezaie P, Dean A. Periventricular leukomalacia, inflammation and white matter lesions within the developing nervous system. *Neuropathology* 2002;22:106–32

21. Volpe JJ. Hypoxic–ischemic encephalopathy: neuropathology and pathogenesis, clinical aspects. In *Neurology of the Newborn*. 4th edn. Philadelphia: W.B. Saunders, 2001:296–394

22. Pooh RK, Maeda K, Pooh KH, *et al.* Sonographic assessment of fetal brain morphology. *Prenat Neonat Med* 1999;4:18–38

23. Yamamoto N, Utsu M, Serizawa M, *et al.* Neonatal periventricular leukomalacia preceded by fetal periventricular echodensity. *Fetal Diag Ther* 2000;15:198–208

24. Wakai S, Arai T, Nagai M. Congenital brain tumors. *Surg Neurol* 1984;21:597–609

25. Volpe JJ. Brain tumors and vein of Galen malformation. In *Neurology of the Newborn*. 4th edn. Philadelphia: W.B. Saunders, 2001:841–56

26. Sherer DM, Abramowicz JS, Eggers PC, Metlay LA, *et al.* Prenatal ultrasonographic diagnosis of intracranial teratoma and massive craniomegaly with associated high-output cardiac failure. *Am J Obstet Gynecol* 1993;168:97–9

Index